Charting

made **Incredibly Easy!** ™

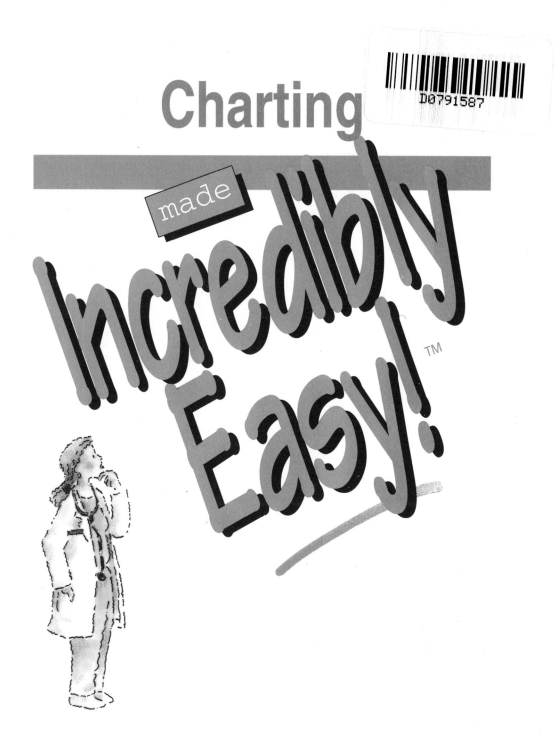

Springhouse Corporation
Springhouse, Pennsylvania

Staff

Senior Publisher
Matthew Cahill

Clinical Director
Judith A. Schilling McCann, RN, MSN

Art Director
John Hubbard

Senior Editor
Michael Shaw

Clinical Editors
Clare Brabson, RN, BSN (project manager);
Carla Roy, RN, BSN, Marybeth Morrell, RN,
CCRN, Theresa P. Fulginiti, RN, BSN, CEN

Editors
Mary Lou Ambrose, Patricia Wittig

Copy Editors
Cynthia C. Breuninger (manager),
Mary T. Durkin, Brenna H. Mayer

Designers
Arlene Putterman (associate art director),
Matie Patterson (assistant art director),
Lorraine Lostracco (book designer),
Joseph Clark, Mary Ludwicki

Illustrator
Bot Roda

Typography
Diane Paluba (manager), Joyce Rossi
Biletz, Phyllis Marron, Valerie Rosenberger

Manufacturing
Deborah Meiris (director), T.A. Landis,
Otto Mezei

Production Coordinator
Stephen P. Hungerford, Jr.

Editorial Assistants
Beverly Lane, Mary Madden

Indexer
Sally Lawther

Printed in the United States of America.

IECH-011297

℞ A member of the Reed Elsevier plc group

Library of Congress Cataloging-in-Publication Data

Charting made incredibly easy.
    p. cm.
    Includes index.

    1. Nursing records. I. Springhouse Corporation.
[DNLM: 1. Nursing Records. 2. Nursing Process
3. Documentation—nurses' instruction   WY 100.5
C486 1997]
    RT50.C483 1997
    610.73—dc21
    DNLM/DLC
    ISBN 0-87434-934-6 (alk. paper)
                                                97-36360
                                                CIP

Contents

Contributors and consultants

Dorothy T. Arnold, RN, BSN
Education Coordinator
Staff Development
Neshaminy Manor Home
Doylestown, Penn.

Nancy Cirone, RN,C, MSN, CDE
Director of Education, Bucks County and
Parkview Hospitals
Allegheny University Hospitals
Warminster, Penn.

Marie S. DeStefano, RN, MS, OCN
Administrative Director
Delaware County Memorial Hospital
Drexel Hill, Penn.

Elizabeth Heum, RN, BA, BS
School Nurse
South Burlington (Vt.) High School

Cynthia Lange Ingham, RN, BSN
Public Health Nursing Specialist
Vermont Department of Health
Burlington

Virginia Lee, RN, MS, MBA
Associate Professor
Northern Virginia Community College
Annandale

Robert Rauch
Medical Economics Manager
Amgen, Inc.
Maple Glen, Penn.

Foreword

As nursing's role in health care has expanded, nurses have taken on greater responsibility in charting care. Now, it's true that some nurses take a dim view of this aspect of their profession. For example, consider the viewpoint of my friend at right:

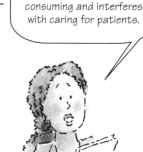

Charting is time consuming and interferes with caring for patients.

Well, I'd like to respond to this viewpoint in simple and straightforward terms: Wake up and smell the coffee!

Charting is every bit as important as other professional nursing responsibilities. First and foremost, you can't separate good patient care from good charting. After all, charting is your official communication link with all other members of the health care team; establishing continuity of care depends on the quality of your documentation. Good charting also provides:
• the most reliable method for substantiating your professional activities
• your first line of defense against malpractice or negligence lawsuits
• crucial data used by your employer for obtaining reimbursement for services you provide to patients
• important information for licensing, accreditation, and efforts to improve the quality of health care.

Unfortunately, until now, books written to help you improve your documentation skills suffer from one essential problem — they're rather dull. However, you're holding a book that represents a revolutionary breakthrough. Leave it to the clinical experts at Springhouse to create a charting book that you'll actually *enjoy* reading. Believe it or not, *Charting Made Incredibly Easy* is delightful as well as full of useful information. Just look inside and you'll be convinced that *Charting Made Incredibly Easy* is unlike any other book on this topic. I can sum up the difference between *Charting Made Incredibly Easy* and other documentation references in four short words: This book is fun.

Part I of *Charting Made Incredibly Easy* discusses charting basics in crystal clear terms. You'll find easy-to-understand information about the medical record, the nursing process, and legal and professional requirements. After covering these fundamental topics, you'll find information on how to develop a solid plan of care and gain new understanding of the different charting systems in use today.

Part II tells you how to chart in specific health care settings, such as acute care, home care, and long-term care and rehabilitation.

Part III provides guidelines for enhancing your charting skills and for avoiding legal pitfalls that can place your career in jeopardy. The final chapter provides detailed instructions for charting specific patient care procedures.

Within each chapter, you'll find many special features to enhance your understanding, expedite your charting, and make learning enjoyable. Each chapter begins with an at-a-glance summary of key topics. Numerous checklists make it easy to spot the most important points. There are even cartoons poking gentle fun at the documentation burden in contemporary health care. A *Quick quiz* at the end of each chapter helps you assess what you've learned. Special logos throughout each chapter alert you to essential information:

Art of the chart alerts you to filled-in forms with key points clearly highlighted. These forms will help you understand exactly how to chart in a wide variety of clinical situations.

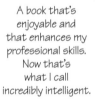

A book that's enjoyable and that enhances my professional skills. Now that's what I call incredibly intelligent.

Advice from the experts offers pointers, tips, and guidelines galore. Learn how to make your charting precise, patient-focused, and litigation-proof.

In sum, enhancing your charting skills is crucial to the well-being of your patients and your career. Becoming familiar with *Charting Made Incredibly Easy* will help you chart efficiently with improved detail and accuracy. In the process, you may gain a fresh perspective on an aspect of practice that all too often is looked upon as drudgery. Hopefully, after you've enjoyed this useful reference for a while, you'll develop a renewed appreciation for *good writing* as a vital skill for practicing the profession of nursing.

Carol L. Schaffer, RN, MSN, JD, MBA
President and Chief Executive Officer
CCF Health Care Ventures, Inc.
Cleveland

Part I

Charting basics

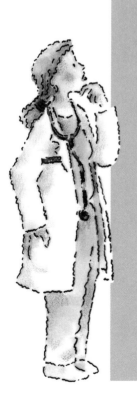

Understanding charting

Just the facts

In this chapter, you'll learn:

♦ why charting matters

♦ how a medical record is organized

♦ the benefits of computer charting.

A look at charting

Charting — or documentation — is the process of preparing a complete record of a patient's care. Accurate, detailed charting shows the extent and quality of the care you've provided, the outcome of that care, and treatment and education that the patient still needs.

Proper charting is important for many reasons. One of the most compelling reasons for you to develop good charting practices is to establish your professional responsibility and accountability.

But, first and foremost, charting is a vital tool for communication among health care team members. Frequently, decisions, actions, and revisions related to the patient's care are based on charting from various team members. A well prepared medical record shows the high degree of collaboration among health care team members.

The information that's documented by team members must be easily retrievable and readable as well. That's because a patient's medical record may be read by a wide audience, including:
• other members of the health care team
• reviewers from accrediting, certifying, and licensing organizations
• quality-improvement monitors
• peer reviewers

- Medicare and insurance company reviewers
- researchers and teachers
- lawyers and judges.

A short history of charting

In the past, charting consisted of cursory observations, such as *patient ate well* or *patient slept well.* The chief purpose of these documents was to show that the doctor's orders and the facility's policies had been followed and that the patient had received the proper care.

In the 19th century, the British nurse Florence Nightingale paved the way for modern nursing documentation. In the book, *Notes on Nursing,* she stressed the importance of training nurses to gather patient information in a clear, concise, organized manner. As her theories gained acceptance, nurses' perceptions and observations about patient care gained credence and respect. More than a century later, in the 1970s, nurses began creating their own vocabulary for documentation based on nursing diagnoses.

Role of charting

Accurate nursing documentation is important for many reasons. Here are nine of them:

It's a mode of communication among health care professionals.

It's checked in health care evaluations.

It's legal evidence that protects you.

It's used to aid research and education.

It helps facilities obtain accreditation and licenses.

It's used to justify reimbursement requests.

It's used to develop improvements in the quality of care.

It indicates compliance with your nurse practice act.

It establishes professional accountability.

Communication

Patients are cared for by many people who work different shifts, and these various caregivers may speak with each other infrequently. The medical record is the main source of information and communication among nurses, doctors, physical therapists, social workers, and other caregivers. Today, nurses are often considered managers of care as well as practitioners, and nurses usually document the most information. Everyone's notes are important, however, because together they present a complete picture of the patient's care.

As health care facilities continue to streamline and redesign care delivery systems, tasks that were historically performed by nurses are now being assigned to multiskilled workers. To deliver highly specialized care, each caregiver must provide accurate, thorough information and be able to interpret what others have written about a patient. Then each can use this information to plan future patient care.

Health care evaluation

When health care is evaluated by other members of the health care team, reviewers, insurance companies, Medicare representatives, lawyers, or judges, accurate documentation is one way to prove that you're providing high-quality care. Complete documentation is both a record of what you do for your patient and written evidence that this care is necessary. It's also a record of your patient's response to your care and any changes you make in his care plan.

Let's see your chart, please.

Legal protection

On the legal side, accurate documentation shows that the care you provide meets the patient's needs and expressed wishes. It also proves that you're following the accepted standards of nursing care mandated by the law, your profession, and your health care facility.

The evidence speaks for itself

How and what you document can determine whether you or your employer wins or loses a legal dispute. Medical records are used as evidence in cases involving disability, personal injury, and mental competency. Poor documentation is the pivotal issue in many malpractice cases. In addition, proper documentation communicates crucial clinical information to caregivers so they make fewer errors.

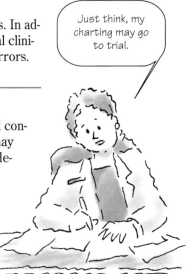

Just think, my charting may go to trial.

Research and education

Documentation also provides data for research and continuing education. For example, medical records may be studied by researchers and nurse educators to determine the validity of nursing diagnoses. They may also be used to gauge how patient teaching affects compliance; the patient's educational level and barriers to learning are noted, as is an assessment of how well he followed the treatment regimen.

On the flip side

Just as documentation is used in research, research studies can be used to improve charting practices. For example, studies may uncover charting errors in the medical record, thereby pointing out the need for continuing education programs for health care providers.

Accrediting and licensing

For a facility to remain accredited, caregivers must document care that reflects the care standards set by national organizations, such as the American Nurses Association and the Joint Commission on Accreditation of Healthcare Organizations (JCAHO). Some states also require facilities to be licensed; licensing laws, in turn, require each facility to establish policies and procedures for operation.

A facility's accreditation and licensure may be jeopardized by substandard documentation. When a facility is cited for having poor documentation or doesn't meet set standards, a warning is given and a target date is set for the facility to make necessary changes and corrections. A facility may lose its license if this isn't accomplished.

Quality is key

In effect, accreditation is evidence that a facility provides quality care and is qualified to receive federal funds. The federal government works with state accrediting organizations to make sure facilities are eligible to receive

Medicare reimbursement. Accreditation and reimbursement eligibility require documentation that accurately reflects the care provided to patients. Good charting demonstrates that facility and state nursing policies were followed.

Getting what they deserve

How do officials of accrediting organizations decide if a facility should be accredited? They look at the facility's structure and function. They also conduct surveys and audits of patient records and medical records to see if care meets the required standards.

Quality and consistency

Officials review charts and files to ensure that good charting is done. For example, in a case where physical restraints were used, officials may ask, "Is there a form for charting the correct use of patient restraints?" and, "Does the documentation in the charts show that restraints were used correctly?" Proper charting reflects the quality of care provided and the facility's accountability.

Accrediting organizations also regularly survey and audit records to make sure the standard of care is consistent throughout a facility. For example, a woman who is recovering from anesthesia after a cesarean birth should expect to receive the same monitoring in the labor and delivery suite as she would in the postanesthesia unit. JCAHO inspectors review the documentation of both departments to ensure that a uniform standard of care is given and documented.

Most accrediting organizations have similar standards for documentation. For example, each patient's medical record must contain the following:
• an assessment
• a care plan
• medical orders
• progress notes
• a discharge summary.

Some organizations spell out the information each of these forms must contain. In these cases, the nurse-manager must write and implement guidelines that meet these requirements.

My charting reflects the quality of my patient care.

Reimbursement

Reimbursement depends heavily on accurate nursing documentation. For example, many hospitals today use elaborate electronic dispensing carts to keep track of supplies. Nursing documentation has to justify the use of these supplies in order to be reimbursed for them.

It's payback time...or is it?

Charting is also used to determine the amount of reimbursement a facility receives. The federal government, for example, uses a prospective payment system based on diagnosis-related groups (DRGs) to determine Medicare reimbursements. In other words, they pay a fixed amount for a particular diagnosis. For a facility to receive payment, the patient's medical record at discharge must contain the correct DRG codes and show that he received the proper care, including appropriate patient teaching and discharge planning.

Most insurance companies likewise base reimbursements on a prospective payment system, and they usually don't reimburse for unskilled nursing care. They pay for skilled medical and nursing care only. For example, they compensate nurse practitioners and home health care nurses for skilled care, which includes assessing a patient's condition, creating a care plan, and following a strict treatment regimen.

Examinations aren't just for patients

Before reimbursing, an examiner studies the patient's medical record to decide whether he needed and received skilled nursing care. The examiner may request copies of the patient's monthly bills and look at documented progress notes, especially if the intensity, frequency, and cost of the care increased.

Examiners also check for inconsistencies in charting, such as a discrepancy between the treatment ordered and the one provided. If the discrepancy isn't explained adequately, the insurer may deny payment.

Preventing premature discharge

Besides keeping a facility from getting reimbursed, faulty documentation can keep patients from getting the care they need. For example, an insurer might deny payment to a home health care agency if the nurse's charting doesn't prove that home visits were necessary. If that happens, home health care may be discontinued prematurely.

My charting may be monitored and evaluated by quality improvement committee members.

Quality improvement

Individual states and the JCAHO require all health care facilities to regularly monitor, evaluate, and seek ways to improve the quality of care for their patients. In each facility, a committee of doctors, nurses, pharmacists, administrators, and other employees gets together to develop quality improvement measures.

Committee members then implement the measures, analyze the improvements, and report their findings to the facility's board of trustees.

Multidisciplinary committee members also develop methods to assess the structure, process, and outcome of patient care. One way to implement these methods is to monitor and evaluate the content of medical records.

Up to snuff?

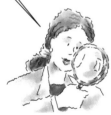

A focus group may investigate ways to improve the quality of care.

What if the care described in a medical record doesn't meet an established standard? Quality improvement committee members must then decide how to correct this problem. They may assign a focus group to investigate ways to do this.

The focus group may recommend changes in the facility's policies, procedures, or documentation forms in an effort to improve patient care. For example, many facilities have been cited in court for lack of documentation when physical restraints were used. As a result, some facilities have developed forms to document restraint orders from doctors. These may be used in court as proof that the facility's policy was followed and that restraints were needed.

Nurse practice acts

Nurse practice acts are state laws spelling out what duties nurses can perform in that state. State nurse practice acts are revised frequently; when nurse practice acts change, charting requirements often change as well. With laws and regulations in a constant state of flux, you must be especially meticulous about charting your care to show compliance with standards.

Accountability

Accurate nursing documentation is evidence that you acted as required or ordered. Accountability means you comply with the charting requirements of your health care facility, professional organizations, and state law.

Types of medical records

Medical records are kept for virtually every person who steps through the door of a health care facility. That's a lot of assessment forms, flow sheets, and nursing diagnosis lists to fill out. How do you deal with this?

An insightful record

Many nurses try to create order in medical records by organizing patient data by category. But this emphasizes form instead of content. *Remember: A medical record isn't just a summary of illness and recovery. It's an insightful record of a patient's care and potential patient care problems.*

Forms are your friends

You can think of the medical record as an ally in your organization efforts. It's a place to organize your thoughts about patient care and record your actions. Used properly, it can help you save time, identify problem areas, plan better patient care, and avoid litigation. (See *Tips for fast, faultless charting,* page 10.)

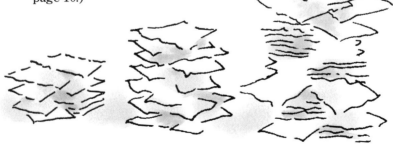

Although every medical record provides evidence of the quality of patient care, all records aren't alike. Some are organized by a source-oriented narrative method, some by a problem-oriented method, and others by variations of these two.

Source-oriented narrative method

With the source-oriented narrative method, caregivers (the source) from each discipline record information in a separate section of the medical record.

On the down side

This traditional method of documentation has several serious drawbacks: Because charting is done in various parts of the record, information is disjointed, topics aren't always clearly identified, and information is difficult to retrieve. This keeps team members from getting a complete picture of the patient's care and causes breakdowns in communication.

Let's get together

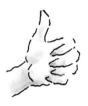

Collaborations among team members who use source-oriented narrative charting are more easily documented if everyone writes on the same progress notes. For example, doctors', nurses', and respiratory therapists' progress notes can be combined into what may be called patient progress notes. These serve as the primary source of reference and communication among health care team members.

Problem-oriented method

A problem-oriented medical record contains baseline data obtained from all departments involved in a patient's care. The problem-oriented charting method is based on the patient's complaints and illness. Data include the following:
• the patient's health history, including his medical, social, and emotional status
• other initial assessment findings
• diagnostic test results.
    The problem-oriented record also contains:
• a problem list
• a care plan for each problem
• progress notes.

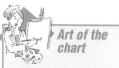
Art of the chart

Tips for fast, faultless charting

When you document, you must record information quickly without sacrificing accuracy. Here are some actions you can take to help you accomplish these two goals:
• Follow the nursing process.
• Use nursing diagnoses.
• Use flow sheets.
• Document at bedside.
• Individualize your charting.
• Don't repeat information (this could lead to errors).
• Sign off with your initials.
• Don't document for other caregivers.
• Use computerized documentation.
• Use fax machines.

The problem list is distilled from baseline data and used to construct a care plan. (See *Got a problem?*)

The care plan in a problem-oriented medical record addresses each of the patient's problems, which are routinely updated both in the plan and in the progress notes. (See *A close look at a medical record*, page 12.)

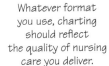

Whatever format you use, charting should reflect the quality of nursing care you deliver.

Other medical record formats

Some facilities modify the source-oriented or problem-oriented method of documentation to suit their needs. If your facility does this, you're in a position to influence the type and style of documentation you use in medical records.

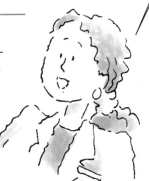

Designer documentation

For example, home health care nurses have created many specialized documentation forms —

Art of the chart

Got a problem?

The chart below shows a nursing problem list for a patient with pancreatitis.

#	Date	Problem statement	Initials	Resolved
1	11/4/91	Fluid volume deficit related to vomiting	C.B.	
2	11/4/91	Pain related to physiologic factors	C.B.	
3	11/4/91	Nutrition alteration: Less than body requirements related to inability to digest nutrients	C.B.	
4	11/4/91	Tissue perfusion alteration (GI) related to decreased cellular exchange	C.B.	
5	11/6/91	Ineffective individual coping related to situational crisis	B.A.	

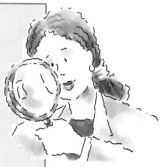

A close look at a medical record

Although each health care facility has its own system for keeping medical records, most records contain the documents described below:

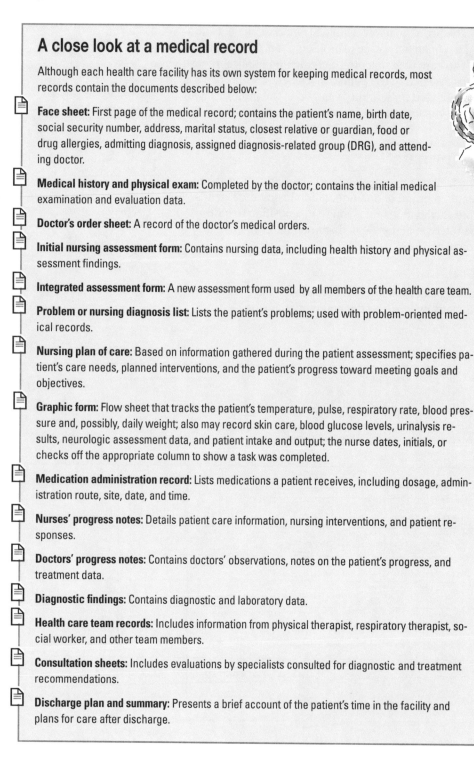

Face sheet: First page of the medical record; contains the patient's name, birth date, social security number, address, marital status, closest relative or guardian, food or drug allergies, admitting diagnosis, assigned diagnosis-related group (DRG), and attending doctor.

Medical history and physical exam: Completed by the doctor; contains the initial medical examination and evaluation data.

Doctor's order sheet: A record of the doctor's medical orders.

Initial nursing assessment form: Contains nursing data, including health history and physical assessment findings.

Integrated assessment form: A new assessment form used by all members of the health care team.

Problem or nursing diagnosis list: Lists the patient's problems; used with problem-oriented medical records.

Nursing plan of care: Based on information gathered during the patient assessment; specifies patient's care needs, planned interventions, and the patient's progress toward meeting goals and objectives.

Graphic form: Flow sheet that tracks the patient's temperature, pulse, respiratory rate, blood pressure and, possibly, daily weight; also may record skin care, blood glucose levels, urinalysis results, neurologic assessment data, and patient intake and output; the nurse dates, initials, or checks off the appropriate column to show a task was completed.

Medication administration record: Lists medications a patient receives, including dosage, administration route, site, date, and time.

Nurses' progress notes: Details patient care information, nursing interventions, and patient responses.

Doctors' progress notes: Contains doctors' observations, notes on the patient's progress, and treatment data.

Diagnostic findings: Contains diagnostic and laboratory data.

Health care team records: Includes information from physical therapist, respiratory therapist, social worker, and other team members.

Consultation sheets: Includes evaluations by specialists consulted for diagnostic and treatment recommendations.

Discharge plan and summary: Presents a brief account of the patient's time in the facility and plans for care after discharge.

including an initial assessment form, problem list, day-visit sheet, and discharge summary — to reflect the unique services and the essential quality of care they provide. These forms meet their charting needs while complying with state and federal laws and other regulations. (See *Specialized forms.*)

Art of the chart

Specialized forms

This form was developed by RNs, LPNs, and Mental Health Technicians to target the essential elements of charting on their unit.

Behavioral Services Department

Patient Stamp

SIP _I _II _III
[ ] Pt suicidal
[ ] Pt has plan
[ ] Pt is homicidal
[ ] Pt has plan
Affect _____ flat _____
ADL's __ good __ fair ✓ poor
[✓] Pt made contact
[ ] did not make contact
[✓] Pt attended groups
[ ] did not attend groups
[✓] attended some groups
[ ] Pt compliant with SA program
[ ] Pt socializing with peers
[ ] Pt seclusive/withdrawn
[✓] Pt select interacting
[ ] Pt hostile
[✓] Pt ate breakfast _10%_
[✓] Pt ate lunch _25%_
[ ] Pt ate snack
[✓] Pt had BM
[ ] No BM _____ days
[ ] action taken_____
[✓] Dual Diagnosis track
[ ] compliant with SA groups
[✓] med. seeking
[ ] consultation completed

NURSE'S NOTES

Date: 12/11/91

72 hr notice
Time _____
Dr. notified _____
Notice rescinded _____

This checklist targets key assessment and evaluation parameters.

7-3 SHIFT   ☐ **Admission Note**   ☑ **Nursing Problem**

12/11/91 0930. Ineffective individual coping related to alcohol abuse and wife leaving him. Denies that alcohol is a problem, states "I only drank more lately because she left me. I drink because I want to, not because I have to." M. Carson, RN
12-11-91 1400. Went to 1100 A.A. meeting, stated "I don't want to be with other people now." Went to room to rest. —————————— M. Carson, RN

Computer charting

Computerized charting is becoming increasingly popular for completing medical records from admission through discharge. The following are some of the benefits provided by computerized documentation:
• It promotes standardization.
• Legibility problems that accompany handwritten entries are eliminated.
• Fewer errors may be made.
• It leads to decreased recording time and costs.
• Communication among team members is aided.
• It allows easier access to medical data for education, research, and quality improvement.

Information filed on computers includes nursing care plans, progress notes, medication records, records of vital signs, intake and output sheets, and patient classifications. Some hospitals even have bedside computers for quick data entry and access. (See *Super-successful automated charting*.)

Super-successful automated charting

To be effective, an automated charting system must be able to:
• record and send data to the appropriate department
• adapt easily to the health care facility's needs
• display highly selective information on command
• provide easy access and retrieval for all trained personnel.

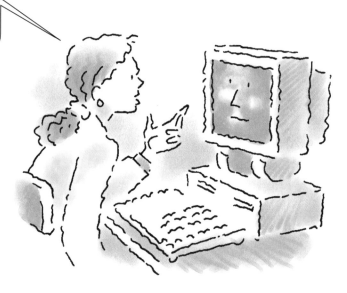

Now, you're supposed to make charting easier.

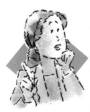

Quick quiz

1. The main drawback to source-oriented narrative records is:
   A. they're problem oriented.
   B. a baseline assessment is needed.
   C. each discipline records information on a separate section of the record.

Answer: C. This type of charting causes communication breakdowns because information is disjointed and hard to retrieve, topics aren't always clearly identified, and team members can't easily get a complete picture of the patient's care.

2. One thing that is not a benefit of charting on a computer is:
   A. there are fewer forms to fill out.
   B. it promotes standardization.
   C. legibility is improved.

Answer: A. Computers can decrease the use of bulky paper files because they store information permanently for easy access and retrieval. However, you still have to complete all the required forms.

3. The JCAHO regulates standards of care in order to:
   A. make sure that all nurses use the same charting system.
   B. ensure quality patient care.
   C. ensure subjective documentation.

Answer: B. To meet JCAHO standards, facilities must uphold certain levels of quality in patient care.

4. Nursing documentation as we know it today was first used in:
   A. the 1970s.
   B. the 19th century.
   C. the 18th century.

Answer: B. Florence Nightingale established modern nursing documentation in the 19th century.

5. The part of the medical record that can be used as evidence in court is:

    A. the care plan.

    B. the medical orders.

    C. the entire record.

Answer: C. The entire medical record is a legal document that's admissible in court.

Scoring

☆☆☆ If you answered all five items correctly, fantastic! You're clear, concise, and consistent — a charting champion!

☆☆ If you answered three or four correctly, dandy! Your documentation definitely deserves to be accredited.

☆ If you answered fewer than three correctly, don't worry. With a little review your recording will reap regular reimbursement!

The nursing process

A look at the nursing process

The nursing process is a problem-solving approach to nursing care. It's a systematic method for determining the patient's health problems, devising a plan of care to address them, implementing the plan, and evaluating the effectiveness of the care.

The nursing process emerged in the 1960s, as team health care came into wider practice and nurses were increasingly called on to define their specific roles. The roots of the nursing process can be traced to World War II, however, when technology, medical advances, and a growing need for nurses began to change the nursing profession.

The nursing process is a six-step path from assessment to evaluation.

Six phases

The nursing process consists of six distinct phases:

☝ assessment

✌ nursing diagnosis

outcome identification

planning

implementation

evaluation.

These six phases are dynamic and flexible and they often overlap. Together, they resemble the steps that many other professions rely on to identify and correct problems.

Assessment

The first step in the nursing process — assessment — begins when you first see a patient. Assessment continues throughout the patient's hospitalization as you obtain more information about his changing condition.

During assessment, you collect relevant information from various sources and analyze it to form a complete picture of your patient. As you collect this information, you need to document it accurately for two reasons:
• It guides you through the rest of the nursing process, helping you formulate nursing diagnoses, expected outcomes, and nursing interventions.
• It serves as a vital communication tool for other team members and as a baseline for evaluating a patient's progress.

The information that you gather at the first patient contact may indicate that the patient needs a broader or more detailed assessment such as a nutritional assessment. (See *Assessing nutritional status.*)

Further assessment depends on the following.
• the patient's diagnosis
• the care setting
• the patient's consent to treatment
• the care the patient is seeking
• the patient's response to previous care.

In your initial assessment, take into account the patient's immediate and emerging needs, including not only his physical needs but psychological and social concerns as well. The initial assessment helps you determine what care the patient needs and sets

> The assessment data I collect establish the basis for the rest of the nursing process.

the stage for further assessments. Remember that a patient's family, culture, and religion are important factors in the patient's response to illness and treatment.

Begin your assessment by collecting a health history and conducting a physical examination.

Health history

The health history includes physical, psychological, cultural, and psychosocial data. It's the main source of information about the patient's health status and guides the physical examination that follows.

A nursing history is different from a medical history. A medical history guides diagnosis and treatment of illness; a nursing history focuses holistically on the human response to illness.

The nursing history you collect helps you to:
• plan health care
• assess the impact of illness on the patient and members of his family
• evaluate the patient's health education needs
• initiate discharge planning.

Getting started

Although nurses conduct health histories in different ways, all interviews must progress in a logical sequence and be an organized record of the patient's response.

Before conducting the health history, consider the patient's ability to participate. If he's sedated, confused, hostile, angry, dyspneic, or in pain, ask only the most essential questions. Then perform an in-depth interview later. In the meantime, ask family members or close friends to provide some information.

Get off on the right foot by finding a quiet, private space where the patient feels as comfortable and relaxed as possible. Ask another nurse to cover your other patients so you won't be interrupted. This reassures the patient that you're interested in what he says and that you'll keep the information confidential. (See *Health history do's and don'ts,* page 20.)

Compressing time

Finding time to conduct a thorough patient history can be hard. But a few strategies can help you keep interview time to a minimum without sacrificing quality. (See *Health history in a hurry,* page 21.)

Assessing nutritional status

As part of the admission assessment, the answers to some questions automatically call for another discipline to be consulted. An example is in the nutrition section.

With the following questions, one "no" requires a nutritional consult:

☑ Do you have sufficient funds to buy food?

☑ Do you have access to a food market?

☑ Are you able to shop, cook, and feed yourself?

With the following questions, one "yes" requires a nutritional consult:

☑ Do you have an illness or condition that made you change the amount or kind of food you ate?

☑ Do you have any dental or mouth problems that made it difficult for you to chew or swallow food?

☑ Do you need help in getting to a food market?

☑ Have you lost or gained 10 lb within the last 6 months without trying?

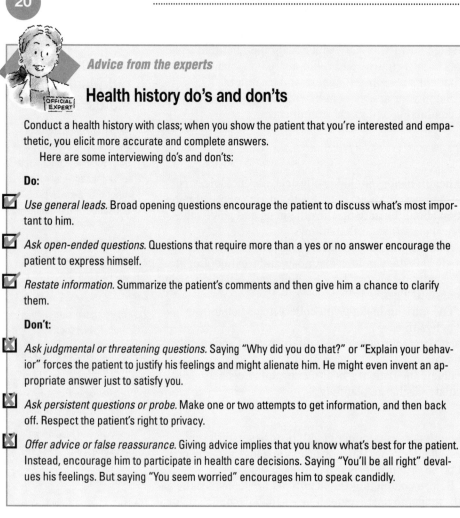

Advice from the experts

Health history do's and don'ts

Conduct a health history with class; when you show the patient that you're interested and empathetic, you elicit more accurate and complete answers.

Here are some interviewing do's and don'ts:

Do:

☑ *Use general leads.* Broad opening questions encourage the patient to discuss what's most important to him.

☑ *Ask open-ended questions.* Questions that require more than a yes or no answer encourage the patient to express himself.

☑ *Restate information.* Summarize the patient's comments and then give him a chance to clarify them.

Don't:

☒ *Ask judgmental or threatening questions.* Saying "Why did you do that?" or "Explain your behavior" forces the patient to justify his feelings and might alienate him. He might even invent an appropriate answer just to satisfy you.

☒ *Ask persistent questions or probe.* Make one or two attempts to get information, and then back off. Respect the patient's right to privacy.

☒ *Offer advice or false reassurance.* Giving advice implies that you know what's best for the patient. Instead, encourage him to participate in health care decisions. Saying "You'll be all right" devalues his feelings. But saying "You seem worried" encourages him to speak candidly.

Sometimes an interview isn't even necessary — you can simply ask the patient to complete a questionnaire about his past and present health status. Then you can quickly and easily document the patient's health history by reviewing the information on the questionnaire and filing it in the patient's chart.

This method is most successful for patients who are to undergo short or elective procedures. The questionnaire can be completed before the patient's admission, which can save you time.

In some acute care settings, modified questionnaires are used to evaluate language and reading problems that the patient may have. The nurse then reviews sections that are completed by the patient.

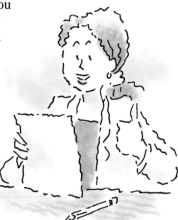

If a questionnaire saves time, I'm all for it!

> **I can't waste time**
>
> ## Health history in a hurry
>
> When you're pressed for time, use the following tips to speed up health history documentation:
>
> - Before the interview, fill in as much information as you can from admission forms, transfer summaries, and the medical history. This avoids duplication of effort. If some information isn't clear, ask the patient for more details. For instance, you might say, "You told Dr. Brown that you sometimes feel like you can't catch your breath. Can you tell me more about when this happens?"
>
> - Check your facility's policy on who may gather assessment data. Maybe you can have an unlicensed nursing assistant or technician collect routine information, such as allergies and past hospitalizations. Remember, though, that reviewing and verifying the information is your responsibility.
>
> - Begin by asking about the patient's chief complaint and the reason he sought medical care. Then, even if the interview is interrupted, you'll still be able to write a care plan.
>
> - Use your facility's nursing assessment documentation form only as a guide to organize information. Ask your patient only pertinent questions from the form.
>
> - Take only brief notes during the interview, so you don't interrupt the flow of conversation. Write detailed notes as soon as possible after the interview. You can always go back to the patient if you need to clarify or verify information.
>
> - Record your findings in concise, specific phrases. Use only approved abbreviations.

Physical examination

The second half of the assessment process is performing a physical examination. Use the following techniques to conduct the examination:
- inspection
- palpation
- percussion
- auscultation.

The objective data you gather during the physical examination may be used to confirm or rule out health problems that were suggested or suspected during the health history. You rely on these findings when you develop a plan of care and in your patient teaching as well. For example, if the patient's blood pressure is high, he may need a sodium-restricted diet and teaching on how to control hypertension.

How detailed should your examination be? That depends on the patient's condition, the clinical setting, and
the policies and procedures established by your health
care facility. The main components of the physical examination include the following:
• height
• weight
• vital signs
• review of the major body systems. (See *Rapid review of
the physical assessment.*)

JCAHO standards

Under the standards of the Joint Commission on Accreditation of Healthcare Organizations (JCAHO), your initial
assessment of the patient should take into consideration
the following:
• physical factors
• psychological and social factors
• environmental factors
• self-care capabilities
• learning needs
• discharge planning needs
• input from the patient's family and friends when appropriate.

Physical factors

Physical factors include the physical examination findings
from your review of the patient's major body systems.

Psychological and social factors

The patient's fears, anxieties, and other concerns about
hospitalization are psychological and social factors. Find
out what support systems the patient has by asking something like, "How does being in the hospital affect your
home situation?" A patient who's worried about his family
might be less able or willing to comply with treatment.

Environmental factors

The patient's home environment affects care needs during
hospitalization and after discharge. Factors to ask about
may include the following:
• where he lives; whether it's a house or an apartment

Advice from the experts

Rapid review of the physical assessment

During a physical examination, your main task is to record the patient's height, weight, and vital signs and review the major body systems. Here's a typical body system review for an adult patient.

Respiratory system
Note the rate and rhythm of respirations, and auscultate the lung fields. Inspect the lips, mucous membranes, and nail beds. Also inspect sputum, noting color, consistency, and other characteristics.

Cardiovascular system
Note the color and temperature of the extremities, and assess the peripheral pulses. Check for edema and hair loss on the extremities. Inspect the neck veins and auscultate for heart sounds.

Neurologic system
Inspect the patient's head for evidence of trauma. Assess his level of consciousness, noting his orientation to person, place, and time and his ability to follow commands. Also assess pupillary reactions. Check extremities for movement and sensation.

Eyes, ears, nose, and throat
Assess the patient's ability to see objects with and without corrective lenses. Assess his ability to hear spoken words clearly. Inspect the eyes and ears for discharge; the nasal mucous membranes for dryness, irritation, and blood; and the teeth for cleanliness. Observe the condition of the oral mucous membranes, and palpate the lymph nodes in the neck.

GI system
Auscultate for bowel sounds in all quadrants. Note abdominal distention or ascites, and assess the condition of the mucous membranes around the anus.

Musculoskeletal system
Assess the range of motion of major joints. Look for swelling at the joints and for contractures, muscle atrophy, or obvious deformity.

Genitourinary and reproductive systems
Note any bladder distention or incontinence. If indicated, inspect the genitalia for rashes, edema, or deformity. (Inspection of the genitalia may be waived at the patient's request or if no dysfunction was reported during the interview.) If indicated, inspect the genitalia for sexual maturity. Also examine the breasts, noting any abnormalities.

Integumentary system
Note any sores, lesions, scars, pressure ulcers, rashes, bruises, or petechiae. Also note the patient's skin turgor.

• whether he has adequate heat, ventilation, hot water, and bathroom facilities
• how many flights of stairs he has to climb; whether the layout of his home poses any hazards
• whether his home is convenient to stores and doctors' offices.

In addition, ask if he uses equipment when performing activities of daily living (ADLs) at home that isn't available in the hospital. Tailor your questions to his condition.

Self-care capabilities

A patient's ability to perform ADLs affects how well he complies with therapy before and after discharge. So assess your patient's ability to eat, wash, dress, use the bathroom, turn in bed, get out of bed, and get around.

Some facilities use an ADL checklist to indicate if a patient can perform these tasks independently or if he needs assistance.

Learning needs

Deciding early what your patient needs to know about his condition leads to effective patient teaching. During the initial assessment, evaluate your patient's knowledge of the disease process, self-care, diet, medications, lifestyle changes, treatment measures, and limitations caused by the disease or treatment.

No yes-or-no answers, please

One way to evaluate your patient's learning needs is to ask open-ended questions, like "What do you know about the medicine you take?" His response will tell you if he understands and complies with his medication regimen or if he needs more teaching.

You also should assess factors that can hinder learning. This can result from:
• the nature of the patient's illness or injury
• the patient's health beliefs
• the patient's religious beliefs
• the patient's educational level
• sensory deficits (such as hearing problems)
• language barriers
• the patient's stress level
• the patient's age
• pain or discomfort.

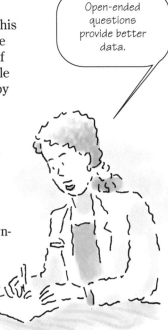

Open-ended questions provide better data.

Discharge planning needs

Discharge planning also should start as soon as possible (in some cases, even before admission), especially if the patient needs help after discharge. Find out where the patient will go after discharge. Is follow-up care accessible?

Art of the chart

Discharge assessment questions

The sample discharge assessment form below is one section of the nursing admission assessment form.

Discharge planning needs

Living arrangements/caregiver: _Sara Smith (patient's daughter)_____

Type of dwelling: Apartment _____ House ✔ Nursing home _____ Boarding home _____ Other _____

Physical barriers in home: No _____ Yes ✔ Explain: _12 step flight of stairs to bathroom and bedroom_____

Access to follow-up medical care: Yes ✔ No _____ Explain: _____

Ability to carry out ADLs: Self-care _____ Partial assistance _____ Total assistance ✔

Needs help with: Bathing ✔ Eating ✔ Ambulation ✔ Other_____

Anticipated discharge destination: Home _____ Rehab _____ Nursing home ✔ Skilled nursing facility _____

Boarding home _____ Other _____

Are community resources — such as visiting nurse services and Meals on Wheels — available where he lives? If not, you need time to help the patient make other arrangements. (See *Discharge assessment questions*.)

Because inpatient lengths of stay have become shorter and patient care has become increasingly complex, nurses need to prioritize their assessment data. (See *Establishing priorities for patient assessment*, page 26.)

Input from family and friends

Another JCAHO requirement is that you obtain assessment information from the patient's family and friends, when appropriate. When you interview someone other than the patient, be sure to document the nature of the relationship. If the interviewee is not a family member, ask about and record the length of time the person has known the patient.

Nursing diagnosis

Your assessment findings form the basis for the next step in the nursing process: the nursing diagnosis. According to the North American Nursing Diagnosis Association, a nursing diagnosis is a clinical judgment about the patient's response to actual or potential health problems or life processes. Nursing diagnoses are used in selecting nursing interventions to achieve outcomes for which the nurse is accountable.

Ingredients of a diagnosis

Each nursing diagnosis describes an actual or potential health problem that a nurse can legally manage. A diagnosis usually has three components:

  the human response or problem — an actual or potential problem that can be affected by nursing care

  related factors — may precede, contribute to, or be associated with the human response

  signs and symptoms — defining characteristics that lead to the diagnosis.

One patient, two types of treatment

Once you become familiar with nursing diagnoses, you'll clearly see how nursing practice and medical practice differ. Although problems are identified in both nursing and medicine, medical and nursing treatment approaches are very different.

The main difference is that doctors are licensed to diagnose and treat illnesses, and nurses are licensed to diagnose and treat the patient's *response* to illness. Nurses also can diagnose the need for patient education, offer comfort and counsel to patients and families, and care for patients until they're physically and emotionally ready to provide self-care.

Emergencies get top billing

Whenever you develop nursing diagnoses, you must prioritize them. Then begin your plan of care with the highest priority. High-priority diagnoses involve emergency or immediate physical care needs.

Intermediate-priority diagnoses involve nonemergency needs, and low-priority diagnoses involve needs that don't directly relate to the patient's illness or prognosis. Maslow's hierarchy of needs can help you set priorities in your plan of care. (See *Maslow's pyramid.*)

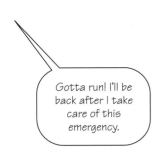

Gotta run! I'll be back after I take care of this emergency.

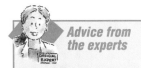

Advice from the experts

Establishing priorities for patient assessment

After the nurse performs an initial assessment, the Joint Commission on Accreditation of Healthcare Organizations requires that she use the information gathered to prioritize her care decisions. To systematically set priorities, follow these steps:

☑ Identify the patient's problems.

☑ Identify the patient's risk for injury.

☑ Identify the patient's need for help with self-care, both in the hospital and following discharge.

☑ Identify the education needs of the patient and members of his family.

Maslow's pyramid

To formulate nursing diagnoses, you must know your patient's needs and values. Of course, physiologic needs — represented by the base of the pyramid in the diagram below — must be met first.

Self-actualization
Recognition and realization of one's potential, growth, health, and autonomy

Self-esteem
Sense of self-worth, self-respect, independence, dignity, privacy, self-reliance

Love and belonging
Affiliation, affection, intimacy, support, reassurance

Safety and security
Safety from physiologic and psychological threat; protection, continuity, stability, lack of danger

Physiologic needs
Oxygen, food, elimination, temperature control, sex, movement, rest, comfort

SELF-ACTUALIZATION
SELF-ESTEEM
LOVE AND BELONGING
SAFETY & SECURITY
PHYSIOLOGIC NEEDS

Outcome identification

The goal of your nursing care is to help your patient reach his highest functional level with minimal risk and problems. If he can't recover completely, your care should help him cope physically and emotionally with his impaired or declining health.

Be realistic

With this in mind, you should identify realistic, measurable expected outcomes and corresponding target dates for your patient. Expected outcomes are goals the patient should reach as a result of planned nursing interventions. Sometimes, a nursing diagnosis requires more than one expected outcome.

Realistically, I expected that outcome.

An outcome can specify an improvement in the patient's ability to function; for example, an increase in the distance he can walk. Or it can specify the correction of a problem such as a reduction of pain. In either case, each outcome calls for the maximum realistic improvement for a particular patient. Once an expected outcome is achieved, it's called a "patient outcome."

Four-part format

An outcome statement consists of four parts:
• the specific behavior that shows the patient has reached his goal
• criteria for measuring that behavior
• the conditions under which the behavior should occur
• when the behavior should occur. (See *Components of an outcome statement*.)

Components of an outcome statement

An outcome statement consists of four elements: behavior, measure, condition, and time.

   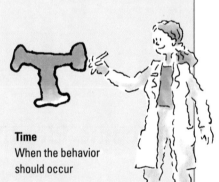

Behavior
A desired behavior for the patient; must be observable

Measure
Criteria for measuring the behavior; should specify how much, how long, how far, and so on

Condition
The conditions under which the behavior should occur

Time
When the behavior should occur

As indicated, the two outcome statements below have these four components.

Ambulate	one flight of stairs	unassisted	by 11/12/91
Demonstrate	measuring radial pulse	before exercising	by 11/12/91

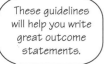

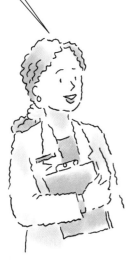

These guidelines will help you write great outcome statements.

Writing outcome statements

Save time when writing outcome statements by choosing your words carefully and being clear and concise. (See *Writing excellent outcome statements.*)

Here are some tips for writing efficient outcome statements:

• *Avoid unnecessary words.* For example, instead of writing *Pt will demonstrate correct wound-care technique by 11/1,* drop the first two words. Everyone knows you're talking about the patient.

• *Use accepted abbreviations.* Refer to your facility's approved abbreviation list. If it uses relative dates (describes the patient's stay in day-long intervals), use abbreviations like *HD1* for hospital day 1 or *POD 2* for postoperative day 2.

• *Make your statements specific. Understand relaxation techniques* doesn't tell you much; how do you observe a patient's understanding? But documenting that the patient should *Practice progressive muscle relaxation techniques unassisted for 15 minutes daily by 4/9* tells you exactly what to look for when assessing the patient's progress.

• *Focus on the patient.* Outcome statements should reflect the patient's behavior, not your intervention. *Medication brings chest pain relief* doesn't say anything about behavior. A correct statement would be *Express relief of chest pain within 1 hour of receiving medication.*

• *Let the patient help you.* A patient who helps write his outcome statements is more motivated to achieve his goals. His input, and his family members', can help you set realistic goals.

• *Consider medical orders.* Don't write outcome statements that ignore or contradict medical orders. For example, before writing *Ambulate 10' unassisted twice a day by 11/9,* make sure that the medical orders don't call for more restricted activity, like bedrest.

• *Adapt the outcome to the circumstances.* Consider the patient's coping ability, age, education, cultural influences, family support, living conditions, socioeconomic status, and anticipated length of stay. Also consider the health care setting. For example, *Ambulates outdoors with assistance for 20 minutes t.i.d by 11/9* is probably unrealistic in a large city hospital.

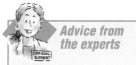

Advice from the experts

Writing excellent outcome statements

The following tips will help you write clear, precise outcome statements:

☑ When writing expected outcomes in your plan of care, always start with a specific action verb that focuses on your patient's behavior. By telling your reader how your patient should *look, walk, eat, drink, turn, cough, speak,* or *stand,* for example, you give a clear picture of how to evaluate progress.

☑ Avoid starting expected outcome statements with *allow, let, enable,* or similar verbs. Such words focus attention on your own and other health team members' behavior — not on the patient's.

☑ With many documentation formats, you won't need to include the phrase *The patient will...* with each expected outcome statement. You will, however, have to specify which person the goals refer to when family, friends, or others are directly concerned.

Planning care

The fourth step of the nursing process is planning. The nursing plan of care is a written plan of action designed to help you deliver quality patient care. The plan of care is based on problems identified during the patient's admission interview. The plan consists of:
• nursing diagnoses
• expected outcomes
• nursing interventions.
    The plan of care usually becomes a permanent part of the patient's record and is used by all members of the nursing team. *Remember: Patients' problems and needs change, so review your plan of care often and modify it if necessary.*

Take three giant steps

Writing a plan of care involves these three steps:
• assigning priorities to the nursing diagnoses
• selecting appropriate nursing interventions to accomplish expected outcomes
• documenting the nursing diagnoses, expected outcomes, nursing interventions, and evaluations. (See *Tips for top-notch care plans.*)

Implementation

Now you're ready to select interventions and implement them, the fifth step of the nursing process. Nursing interventions are actions that you and your patient agree will help him reach the expected outcomes. Base these interventions on the second part of your nursing diagnosis, the related factors.
    For example, with a nursing diagnosis of *Impaired physical mobility related to arthritic morning stiffness,* select interventions that reduce or eliminate the patient's stiffness such as mild stretching exercises. Write at least one intervention for each outcome statement.

Divine intervention

How do you come up with interventions? There are several ways. First, consider interventions that you or your patient have successfully tried before. For example, if the patient's having trouble sleeping in the hospital, and he tells

Advice from the experts

Tips for top-notch care plans

Use either a traditional or standardized method for recording your plan of care. A traditional plan of care is written from scratch for each patient. A standardized plan of care saves time because it's predetermined, based on the patient's diagnosis.

No matter which method you use, follow these tips to write a plan that's accurate and useful:

☑ Write in ink and sign your name.

☑ Use clear, concise language, not vague terms or generalities.

☑ Use standard abbreviations to avoid confusion.

☑ Review all your assessment data *before* selecting an approach for each problem. If you can't complete the initial assessment, immediately write *insufficient information* on your records.

☑ Write an expected outcome and a target date for each problem you identify.

☑ Set realistic initial goals.

☑ When writing nursing interventions, consider what to watch for and how often, what nursing measures to take and how to perform them, and what to teach the patient and family before discharge.

☑ Make each nursing intervention specific.

☑ Make sure your interventions match the resources and capabilities of the staff.

☑ Be creative; include a drawing or an innovative procedure if this makes your directions more specific.

☑ Record all of the patient's problems and concerns so they won't be forgotten.

☑ Make sure your plan is implemented correctly.

☑ Evaluate the results of your plan and discontinue nursing diagnoses that have been resolved. Select new approaches, if necessary, for problems that haven't been resolved.

you that a glass of warm milk helps him get to sleep at home, this could work as an intervention for the expected outcome *Sleep through the night without medication by 11/9.*

You also can pick interventions from standardized plans of care, ask other nurses about interventions they've used successfully, or check nursing journals for ideas. If these methods don't work, try brainstorming with other nurses.

Writing interventions

To help you write interventions clearly and correctly, follow these guidelines:

• *Clearly state the necessary action.* Note how and when to perform the intervention, and include special instructions. *Promote comfort* doesn't say what specific action to take, but *Administer ordered analgesic ½ hour before dressing change* says exactly what to do and when to do it.

• *Make interventions fit the patient.* Consider the patient's age, condition, developmental level, environment, and values. For instance, if he's a vegetarian, don't write an intervention that requires him to eat lean meat to gain extra protein for healing.

• *Keep the patient's safety in mind.* Consider the patient's physical and mental limitations. For instance, before teaching a patient how to give himself medication, be sure he's physically able to do it and that he can remember and follow the regimen.

• *Follow your facility's rules.* For example, if your facility allows only nurses to administer medications, don't write an intervention calling for the patient to *Administer hemorrhoidal suppositories as needed.*

• *Consider other health care activities.* Adjust your interventions when other activities interfere with them. For example, you might want your patient to get plenty of rest on a day when he has several diagnostic tests scheduled.

• *Use available resources.* If your patient needs to learn about his cardiac problem, use your facility's education department, literature from the American Heart Association, and local support groups. Write your intervention to reflect the use of these resources.

Charting interventions

Once you've performed an intervention, record the nature of the intervention, the time you performed it, and the patient's response. Also record other interventions that you performed based on his response and the reasons you performed them. This makes your documentation outcome-oriented.

Document in quadruplicate

Where do you document interventions? That depends on your facility's policy. You can document them on graphic records, on a patient care flow sheet that integrates all nurses' notes for a 1-day period, on integrated or separate nurses' progress notes, and on other specialized documentation forms such as the medication administration record.

Your facility's policies also dictate the style and format of your documentation. You should record interventions when you give routine care, give emergency care, observe changes in the patient's condition, and administer medications.

Evaluation

The current emphasis on evaluating your interventions has changed documentation. Traditional documentation didn't always reflect the end results of nursing care. But today, your progress notes must include an evaluation of your patient's progress toward the expected outcomes you've established in the plan of care.

Charting changes

The latest charting method in town is called *outcomes and evaluation documentation*. It focuses on the patient's response to nursing care and helps you provide high quality, cost-effective care. It's replacing narrative charting and lengthy, handwritten plans of care. (See *Effective evaluation statements*.)

The transition to outcome documentation has been difficult for some nurses. In outcome documentation the nurse is expected to record nursing judgments, not just nursing interventions. Unfortunately, nurses have traditionally been trained not to make judgments. Today, nurses are being asked to gather and interpret data, refer and prioritize care, and document their findings.

The belief that hands-on care is more important than documentation is one reason nurses often focus more on nursing interventions than on documenting patient responses. Outcomes and evaluation documentation compels nurses to focus on patient responses. And when you evaluate the results of your interventions, you help ensure that your plan is working.

Why evaluate?

Evaluation of care gives you a chance to:
• determine if your original assessment findings still apply
• uncover complications

Art of the chart

Effective evaluation statements

The evaluation statements below clearly describe common outcomes. Note that they include specific details of care provided and objective evidence of the patient's response to care.

Response to patient education: *Able to describe the signs and symptoms of hyperglycemia.*

Response to pain medication within 1 hour of administration: *States leg pain decreased from 9 to 6 (on a scale of 1 to 10) 30 minutes after receiving I.M. meperidine.*

Tolerance of change or increase in activity: *Able to ambulate to chair with a steady gait, approximately 10 ', unassisted.*

Tolerance of treatments: *Unable to tolerate removal of O_2; became dyspneic on room air even at rest.*

- analyze patterns or trends in the patient's care and his response to it
- assess the patient's response to all aspects of his care, including medications, changes in diet or activity, procedures, unusual incidents or problems, and teaching
- determine how closely care conforms to established standards
- measure how well you've cared for the patient
- assess the performance of other members of the health care team
- identify opportunities to improve the quality of your care.

Ever-evaluating

Evaluation itself is an ongoing process that takes place whenever you see your patient. However, how often you're required to make evaluations depends on several factors, including where you work.

If you work in an acute care setting, your facility's policy may require you to review plans of care every 24 hours. But if you work in a long-term care facility, the required interval between evaluations may be up to 30 days. In either case, you still should evaluate and revise the plan of care more often if warranted.

Evaluating expected outcomes

Evaluation includes gathering reassessment data, comparing findings with the outcome criteria, determining the extent of outcome achievement (whether the outcome was met, partially met, or not met), writing evaluation statements, and revising the plan of care.

To revise or not to revise

Revision starts with determining whether the patient has achieved the outcomes. If they haven't been fully met and you decide that the problem is resolved, the plan can be discontinued. If the problem persists, continue the plan with new target dates, until the desired status is achieved. If outcomes are partially met or unmet, identify interfering factors, such as misinterpreted information, and revise the plan accordingly. Revision may involve the following:

- clarifying or amending the data base to reflect new information
- reexamining and correcting nursing diagnoses

> Time to evaluate my patient's progress.

• establishing outcome criteria that reflect new information and new or amended nursing strategies
• adding the revised nursing plan of care to the original document
• recording the rationale for the revision in the nurse's progress notes.

I'd better revise my plan.

Documenting evaluation

Evaluation statements should indicate whether expected outcomes were achieved and should list evidence supporting this conclusion. Base these statements on outcome criteria from the plan of care, and use action verbs, such as *demonstrate* or *ambulate*.

Include the patient's response to specific treatments, such as medication administration or physical therapy, and describe the condition under which the response occurred or failed to occur. Document patient teaching and palliative or preventive care as well.

After evaluating the outcome, be sure to record it in the patient's chart with clear statements that demonstrate his progress toward meeting the expected outcomes.

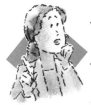

Quick quiz

1. The nursing health history is most accurately described as:
   A. a tool to guide diagnosis and treatment of the illness.
   B. a follow-up to the medical history.
   C. an interview that focuses holistically on the human response to illness.

Answer: C. This is how the nursing health history differs from a medical health history, whose focus is on the diagnosis and treatment of illness.

2. The primary source of assessment information is:
   A. the patient.
   B. past medical records.
   C. the patient's next of kin.

Answer: A. However, if the patient is sedated, confused, hostile, angry, dyspneic, or in pain, you may have to rely initially on family members or close friends to supply information.

3. According to the North American Nursing Diagnosis Association, a nursing diagnosis is a clinical judgment about:
   A. the patient's response to actual or potential health problems or life processes.
   B. the patient's ability to perform activities of daily living.
   C. the patient and family members' emotional response to illness.

Answer: A. A nursing diagnosis is a clinical judgment about the patient's response to actual or potential health problems or life processes.

4. Expected outcomes are defined as:
   A. goals the patient should reach as a result of planned nursing interventions.
   B. what the patient and family ask you to accomplish.
   C. goals a little higher than what the patient can realistically reach to help motivate him.

Answer: A. Expected outcomes are realistic, measurable goals and their target dates.

5. A good way to come up with interventions is by:
   A. asking the doctor.
   B. asking the patient what's worked for him before.
   C. reviewing past medical records.

Answer: B. You can also ask other nurses, check nursing journals, pick interventions from standardized plans of care, or brainstorm.

Scoring

☆☆☆   If you answered all five items correctly, chalk one up to success! You're an avid assessment aficionado!

☆☆   If you answered three or four correctly, document your diligence! You're a dedicated diagnosis devotee!

☆   If you answered fewer than three correctly, keep striving for excellence! Soon you'll be an expert evaluation enthusiast!

Plans of care

Just the facts

In this chapter, you'll learn:

♦ the reasons for writing a plan of care

♦ the differences between traditional and standardized plans of care

♦ the parts of a patient-teaching plan and how to formulate one

♦ about critical pathways and how to use them.

A look at the nursing plan of care

The nursing plan of care is a vital part of documentation. To the health care team, the nursing plan of care is a principal source of information about the patient's problems, needs, and goals. It contains detailed instructions for achieving the goals established for the patient and is used to direct care. It also includes suggestions for solving patient problems and dealing with unexpected complications.

There are four aspects to writing the plan of care:

👆 establishing care priorities (based on assessment data)

✌ identifying expected outcomes

🤟 developing nursing interventions to attain these outcomes and evaluating the patient's responses

🖖 documenting the plan in the format required by your facility.

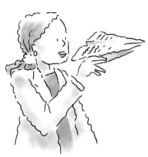

Until 1991, the plan of care wasn't part of the patient's permanent record. It was used by the nursing staff and then discarded when the patient was discharged. Now, the Joint Commission on Accreditation of Healthcare Organizations (JCAHO) requires that the plan of care be permanently integrated into the medical record by written or electronic means.

JCAHO policy changes have also led to greater flexibility when writing plans of care. The commission no longer specifies the format for documenting patient care, so new methods have emerged that can make planning faster and easier.

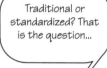

Traditional or standardized? That is the question...

Types of care plans

You may write your plans of care in one of two styles, *traditional* or *standardized.* Whatever approach you use, your plan of care should cover all nursing care from admission to discharge.

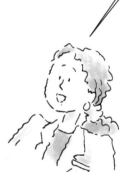

Traditional plan of care

Also called an *individually developed plan of care,* the traditional plan is written from scratch for each patient. After you analyze your assessment data for a patient, you either write the plan by hand or enter it into a computer. (See *It's traditional.*)

The basic form for the traditional care plan varies, depending on the function of this important document in your facility or department. Most forms have three main columns:
• one for nursing diagnoses
• a second for expected outcomes
• a third for interventions.

There may be other columns for the dates when you initiated the plan of care, target dates for expected outcomes, and the dates for review, revisions, and resolutions. Most forms also have a place for you to sign or initial whenever you make an entry or a revision.

Art of the chart

It's traditional

Here's an example of a traditional plan of care. It shows how these forms are typically organized. Remember that a traditional plan is written from scratch for each patient.

Date	Nursing diagnosis	Expected outcomes	Interventions	Revision (initials and date)	Resolution (initials and date)
11/15/91	Breathing pattern, ineffective R/T pain	Respiratory rate stays within +/- 5 of baseline	Assess and record respiratory status q3h		
		ABG levels remain normal	Assess for pain q3h		
		Achieves comfort without depressing respirations	Give pain medication, as ordered p.r.n.		
			Assist patient to a comfortable position		
		Demonstrates correct use of incentive spirometry	Assist patient in using incentive spirometry		
			Teach patient how to splint chest while coughing		
		Auscultation reveals no adventitious breath sounds	Perform chest physiotherapy to aid in mobilizing and removing secretions		
		States understanding of importance of taking deep breaths periodically	Provide rest periods		
			Encourage patient to use incentive spirometry		
		Reports ability to breathe comfortably	Provide oxygen, as ordered		

> Nursing diagnoses, expected outcomes, and interventions are key elements of traditional plans.

Review dates		
Date	Signature	Initials
11/15/91	M. Hopper, RN	MH

Choose your outcome: Short- or long-term

What should you include on the forms? This varies, too. Because shorter hospital stays are more common today, in most health care facilities you're expected to write only short-term outcomes that the patient can reach by the time he's discharged.

However, some facilities — especially long-term care facilities — also want you to chart long-term outcomes for the patient's maximum functioning level. These facilities commonly provide forms with separate spaces for short- and long-term outcomes.

Advantages

Some advantages of the traditional method are:
• It provides a personalized plan for each patient.
• The format allows health care team members and the patient to easily visualize the plan.
• Columns for updates and revisions are clearly delineated.

Disadvantages

The main disadvantage of the traditional method is that it's time-consuming to read and write because lengthy documentation is required.

Standardized plan of care

The standardized plan of care is the most common format used today. A standardized plan eliminates the problems associated with the traditional plan by using preprinted information. This saves documentation time.

Some standardized plans are classified by medical diagnoses or diagnosis-related groups (DRGs); others, by nursing diagnoses. The preprinted information included in a standardized plan of care includes interventions for patients with similar diagnoses and, usually, root outcome statements.

Insist on individuality

Early versions of standardized plans of care didn't allow for differences in patients' needs. However, current versions require you to explain how you've individualized the plan for each patient by adding the following information:
• *"related to" (R/T) statements and signs and symptoms for a nursing diagnosis.* If the form provides a root diagnosis — such as "Pain R/T _____" — you might fill in *inflammation, as exhibited by grimacing, expressions of pain.*
• *time limits for the outcomes.* To a root statement of the goal *Perform postural drainage without assistance,* you might add *for 15 minutes immediately upon awakening in the morning, by 11/12.*

Each patient has unique needs.

• *frequency of interventions.* To an intervention such as *Perform passive range-of-motion exercises,* you might add *twice a day: 1x each in the morning and evening.*
• *specific instructions for interventions.* For the standard intervention *Elevate patient's head,* you might specify *before sleep, on three pillows.*

Computers make combos less cumbersome

When a patient has more than one diagnosis, you have to combine standardized plans of care, which can make records long and cumbersome. However, if your facility uses computerized plans, you can extract only the parts you need from each plan, and then combine them to make one manageable plan. Some computer programs provide a checklist of interventions from which you can select to build your own plan.

Although standardized plans usually include only essential information, most provide space for you to write additional nursing diagnoses, expected outcomes, and interventions. (See *Why stand on tradition? Use a standardized plan,* page 42.)

The upside of standardized plans

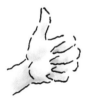

Standardized plans of care offer many advantages, because they:
• require far less writing than traditional plans
• are more legible
• are easier to duplicate and save on microfilm
• make compliance with a facility's policy easier for all members of the health care team: experts, novices, and ancillary staff
• guide you in creating the plan while allowing freedom to adapt it to your patient.

There's always a downside

This method has one main drawback: If you simply check off items on a list or fill in the blanks, you might not individualize the patient's care or document your findings adequately.

Patient-teaching plan

A patient-teaching plan serves several important functions:
• It pinpoints what the patient needs to learn and how he'll be taught.

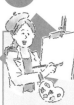

Art of the chart

Why stand on tradition? Use a standardized plan

The standardized plan of care below is for a patient with a nursing diagnosis of decreased cardiac output. To customize it to your patient, complete the diagnosis — including signs and symptoms — and fill in the expected outcomes.

> There's a lot less writing with standardized plans.

Date _12/15/91_

Nursing diagnosis
Tissue integrity impairment related to arterial insufficiency

Target date _12/17/91_

Expected outcome
Attains relief from immediate symptoms: _____ _pain, ulcers, edema_
Voices intent to change aggravating behavior: _____ _will stop smoking immediately_
Maintains collateral circulation: _____ _palpable peripheral pulses, extremities warm_
_____ _and pink with good capillary refill_
Voices intent to follow specific management routines after discharge: _foot care_
_____ _guidelines, exercise regimen as specified by physical therapy department_

Date _12/15/91_

Interventions
- Provide foot care. Administer and monitor treatments according to facility protocols.
- Encourage adherence to exercise regimen as tolerated.
- Educate patient about risk factors and prevention of injury. Refer patient to smoking cessation program.
- Maintain adequate hydration. Monitor I & O _____ _q8h_
- To increase arterial blood supply to the extremities, elevate head of bed _6" to 8"_
- Additional interventions: _____ _Inspect skin integrity q8h_

- It sets criteria for evaluating how well the patient learns.
- It helps all caregivers coordinate their teaching.
- It serves as legal proof that the patient received appropriate instruction and satisfies the requirements of regulatory agencies such as the JCAHO.

Pointers for the perfect plan

To make sure that your teaching plan is as effective as possible, consider carefully what the patient needs to learn, how you'll teach him, and how you'll measure the results. Work closely with the patient, members of his family, and other health care team members to create realistic and attainable goals for your plan. Also provide for follow-up teaching at home.

Be sure to keep your plan flexible. Allow for factors that may interfere with effective teaching, such as a patient's unreceptiveness because of a poor night's sleep or your own daily time constraints.

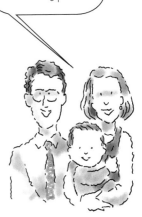

Include family members in your teaching plan.

Parts of the teaching plan

The patient-teaching plan is divided into five sections:

- patient learning needs
- expected learning outcomes
- teaching content
- teaching methods
- teaching tools.

Learning needs

The first step in developing a teaching plan is to identify what your patient needs to learn. Consider what you, the doctor, and other health care team members expect him to learn, as well as what he expects to learn.

Learning outcomes

After you identify the patient's learning needs, you can establish expected learning outcomes. Beginning with your assessment findings, list the topics and strategies that the patient needs to learn to reach the maximum level of health and self-care.

Understand, feel, do

Like other patient care outcomes, expected learning outcomes should focus on the patient and be easy to measure. Learning behaviors and the outcomes you develop fall into three categories:

- *cognitive,* relating to understanding
- *affective,* dealing with attitudes
- *psychomotor,* covering manual skills.

For example, for a patient who's learning to give himself subcutaneous injections, identifying an injection site is a cognitive outcome, coping with the need for injections is an affective outcome, and giving the injection is a psychomotor outcome. (See *Penning precise learning outcomes*.)

Fine-tuning those outcomes

To develop precise, measurable outcomes, decide which evaluation techniques best reveal the patient's progress. For cognitive learning, you might use questions and answers; for psychomotor learning, you might use return demonstration.

To measure affective learning — which can be difficult because changes in attitude develop slowly — you can use several evaluation techniques. For example, to deter-

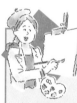

Art of the chart

Penning precise learning outcomes

Learning behaviors fall into three categories: cognitive, psychomotor, and affective. Keeping these categories in mind will help you to write clear, concise learning outcomes. Remember that your outcomes should clarify what you plan to teach, what behavior you expect to see, and what criteria you'll use for evaluating the patient's learning.

Compare the two sets of learning outcomes below.

Well-phrased learning outcomes	Poorly phrased learning outcomes
Cognitive domain	
The patient with heart failure will be able to: • state when to take each prescribed drug. • describe symptoms of heart failure.	The patient with heart failure will be able to • remember his medication schedule. • recognize when his respiratory rate is increased.
Affective domain	
The patient with heart failure will be able to: • report feeling comfortable when breathing. • demonstrate willingness to comply with therapy by keeping scheduled doctor's appointments.	The patient with heart failure will be able to: • adjust successfully to limitations of disease. • realize the importance of seeing his doctor.
Psychomotor domain	
The patient with heart failure will be able to: • demonstrate diaphragmatic pursed-lip breathing. • demonstrate skill in conserving energy while carrying out activities of daily living.	The patient with heart failure will be able to: • take his respiratory rate. • bring in a sputum specimen for laboratory studies.

mine whether a patient has overcome his anxiety about giving himself an injection, try asking him if he still feels anxious. You also can assess his willingness to perform the procedure and observe whether he hesitates or shows other signs of stress while doing it.

Then, write the outcome statement based on the selected evaluation technique. For example, if you select return demonstration as your evaluation technique, an appropriate outcome statement might be *Patient demonstrates skill in carrying out mobility regimen.*

Content

Next, select what to teach the patient to help him achieve the expected outcomes. Be sure to consult with the patient, members of his family, and other caregivers in deciding what to teach. Even if the patient is learning to care for himself, you still should teach a family member how to provide physical and emotional support or how to help the patient remember his care.

Once you've decided what to teach, organize it. Start with the simplest concepts and work toward the more complex ones. This is especially helpful when teaching a patient with little education or one who doesn't learn or listen well.

Methods

Now, select the appropriate teaching methods for your patient. Most of your teaching probably can be done one-on-one. This allows you to learn about your patient, build a relationship with him, and tailor your teaching to his needs.

Other paths to learning

Many different teaching methods work well along with, or instead of, one-on-one teaching. For instance, try incorporating demonstration, practice, and return demonstration in your teaching plan. Role playing can increase your patient's involvement in the plan, as can case studies, which require him to evaluate how someone else with his disorder responds to different situations.

Other methods include self-monitoring, which requires the patient to assess his situation and determine which aspects of his environment or behavior need correction.

You also can conduct group lectures and discussions if several patients require similar instruction.

Tools

Finally, decide what teaching tools will help enhance patient education. (See *Tools for tuning up teaching*.) When choosing your tools, focus on what will work best for the particular patient. For instance, if your patient learns best by watching how something is done, use a videotape of a procedure, a closed-circuit television demonstration, or a slide show.

If the patient prefers a hands-on approach, let him handle the equipment he'll use. If he likes to work interactively at his own pace, try a computerized patient-teaching program. If he learns best by reading, provide written materials.

Tracking down teaching tools

To get the tools you need, consult the staff-development instructors on your unit, your facility's librarian, or staff specialists. If you can't find what you need, call pharmaceutical and medical supply companies in your community. Also, contact national associations and foundations such as the American Cancer Society. These organizations usually have many patient education materials written with the layperson in mind. They also provide pamphlets and brochures in several languages.

Keep the patient's abilities and limitations in mind as you choose teaching tools. For example, before giving him written materials, such as brochures and pamphlets, make sure that he can read and understand them. Keep in mind that the average adult reads at only a seventh-grade level.

It's Greek to me

Likewise, make sure you're aware of any language barriers between you and your patients. Use translators and bilingual aids — such as cards and pamphlets — to overcome these barriers.

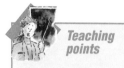

Teaching points

Tools for tuning up teaching

The following list includes teaching materials and methods you can use to optimize your patient's learning.

Teaching materials

- Brochures and pamphlets
- Videotapes
- Closed-circuit television
- Computers
- Equipment being used for his care (for example, syringes, needles, pumps, and IVAC controllers)

Teaching methods

- Role playing
- Return demonstration
- Have student demonstrate understanding by providing instruction to other patients, if appropriate

Documenting the patient-teaching plan

The patient-teaching plan is a key part of the patient's plan of care. By reading it, health care team members can see at a glance what the patient learned and what he still needs to learn. It's also needed by the health care facility to show what quality improvement measures are in progress.

I have to think about this

Constructing individual teaching plans requires time and thought. Fortunately, some facilities have patient education departments that develop and implement standard teaching plans for many common disorders.

Forms, forms, and more forms

There are several different forms for documenting your patient-teaching plan. Many of these incorporate the nursing process as it applies to patient education. (See *Go with the flow sheet,* page 48.)

Just your type

Patient-teaching plans also come in two basic types that are similar to traditional and standardized plans of care. The traditional type provides only the format and requires you to come up with the plan. The standardized type allows you to check off or date steps as you complete them and add or delete information to individualize the plan. It's best suited for patients who need extensive teaching.

Some plans include space for documenting problems that could hinder learning, for comments and evaluations, and for dates and signatures. Or you may need to include this information in your progress notes. No matter which teaching plan you use, this information becomes a permanent part of the patient's medical record.

Critical pathways

A critical pathway is an interdisciplinary care plan that describes assessment criteria, interventions, treatments, and outcomes for specific health-related conditions (usually based on a DRG) across a designated time line.

Think of the pathway as a predetermined checklist describing the tasks you and the patient need to accomplish. In this way, it's similar to a standardized plan of care. However, unlike a plan of care, its focus is multidisciplinary, covering all of the patient's problems, not just those identified during a nursing assessment.

Good teaching requires a good plan.

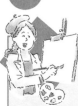

Art of the chart

Go with the flow sheet

Below is the first page of a patient-teaching flow sheet. Flow sheets like this let you quickly and easily tailor your teaching plan to fit your patient's needs.

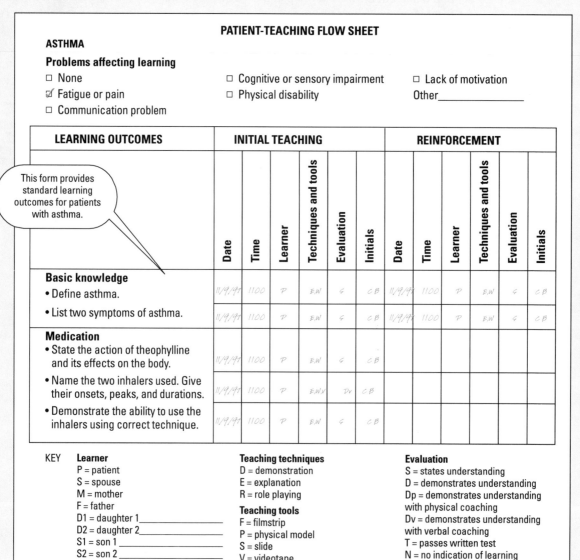

PATIENT-TEACHING FLOW SHEET

ASTHMA

Problems affecting learning

☐ None   ☐ Cognitive or sensory impairment   ☐ Lack of motivation
☑ Fatigue or pain   ☐ Physical disability   Other_____
☐ Communication problem

> This form provides standard learning outcomes for patients with asthma.

LEARNING OUTCOMES	INITIAL TEACHING						REINFORCEMENT					
	Date	Time	Learner	Techniques and tools	Evaluation	Initials	Date	Time	Learner	Techniques and tools	Evaluation	Initials
Basic knowledge												
• Define asthma.	11/9/97	1100	P	E.W	S	C.B	11/9/97	1100	P	E.W	S	C.B
• List two symptoms of asthma.	11/9/97	1100	P	E.W	S	C.B	11/9/97	1100	P	E.W	S	C.B
Medication												
• State the action of theophylline and its effects on the body.	11/9/97	1100	P	E.W	S	C.B						
• Name the two inhalers used. Give their onsets, peaks, and durations.	11/9/97	1100	P	E.W.V	Dv	C.B						
• Demonstrate the ability to use the inhalers using correct technique.	11/9/97	1100	P	E.W	S	C.B						

KEY   **Learner**
          P = patient
          S = spouse
          M = mother
          F = father
          D1 = daughter 1_____
          D2 = daughter 2_____
          S1 = son 1 _____
          S2 = son 2 _____
          O = other_____

Teaching techniques
D = demonstration
E = explanation
R = role playing

Teaching tools
F = filmstrip
P = physical model
S = slide
V = videotape
W = written material

Evaluation
S = states understanding
D = demonstrates understanding
Dp = demonstrates understanding with physical coaching
Dv = demonstrates understanding with verbal coaching
T = passes written test
N = no indication of learning
NE = not evaluated

A documentation tool by any other name

Critical pathways go by many different names: clinical pathways, critical paths, interdisciplinary plans, anticipated recovery plans, care maps, interdisciplinary action plans, and action plans.

Members of the health care team involved in providing care should collaborate to develop each critical pathway. The goals of the critical pathway include:
- achieving expected patient and family outcomes
- promoting professional collaborative practice and care
- ensuring continuity of care
- ensuring appropriate use of resources
- reducing cost and length of stay
- establishing a framework for instituting and monitoring continuous quality improvement.

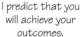

I predict that you will achieve your outcomes.

Practical when predictable

Critical pathways are most useful in specific types of patient care situations. They work well with high-volume cases (meaning the facility cares for a lot of patients with this particular problem) and in situations that have relatively predictable outcomes. Complex situations with unpredictable outcomes normally are not managed with critical pathways.

Love those documentation tools

A critical pathway is a permanent part of the medical record. It provides a consistent assessment and documentation tool for third party payers. It's also used to compare the diagnoses of patients and determine their needs.

Critical pathways cover the key events that must occur before the patient's target discharge date. These events include the following:
- consultations
- diagnostic tests
- treatments
- medications
- procedures
- activities
- diet
- patient teaching
- discharge planning
- achievement of anticipated outcomes.

Charting the path

A critical pathway is usually organized according to categories, such as activity, diet, treatments, medications, patient teaching, and discharge planning. Appropriate categories are determined based on the patient's medical diagnosis. The medical diagnosis also dictates expected length of stay, daily care guidelines, and expected outcomes. Care guidelines are listed under appropriate categories.

The structure of a critical pathway and the categories it contains vary among facilities. Within a facility, the structure and content of critical pathways may vary depending on the specific DRG. (See *Take the critical pathway*.)

Some facilities use nursing diagnoses as the basis for critical pathways, but this is controversial. Critics argue that this format interferes with communication and the coordination of care among non-nursing members of the health care team.

A bundle of benefits

For the most part, critical pathways are a boon for nurses. Here's why:
• They eliminate duplicate charting. The only time you need to write narrative notes is when a standard on the pathway remains unmet or when the patient needs different care than what's written on the form. Most pathways provide a place to document alterations in care.
• With standardized orders or protocols, you can advance the patient's activity level, diet, and treatment regimen without waiting for a doctor's order. Nurses have more freedom to make care decisions.
• Communication improves between members of the health care team because everyone works from the same plan. That's why problems are called *collaborative problems*. The goal is for all members of the team to work together to achieve the desired outcome.
• Quality of care improves because of shared accountability for patient outcomes.
• Patient teaching and discharge planning improves. In facilities where critical pathways are adapted and given to patients, they feel less anxious and are more cooperative because they know what to expect and what is expected of them. Some patients even recover and go home sooner than anticipated.

Art of the chart

Take the critical pathway

At any point in a treatment course, a glance at the critical pathway allows you to compare the patient's progress and your performance as a caregiver with care standards.

The standard critical pathway below outlines care for a patient with a colon resection.

CRITICAL PATHWAY: COLON RESECTION WITHOUT COLOSTOMY

	Patient visit	Presurgery Day-1	Day 0 O.R. Day	Postop Day 1
Assessments	History and physical with breast, rectal, and pelvic exam Nursing assessment	Nursing admission assessment	Nursing admission assessment on TBA patients in holding area Post-op review of systems assessment*	Review of systems assessment*
Consults	Social service consult Physical therapy consult	Notify referring physician of impending admission		
Labs and diagnostics	Complete blood count (CBC) PT/PTT ECG Chest X-ray Chem profile CT ABD w/wo contrast CT pelvis Urine analysis (UA) Ba enema & flex sigmoid-oscopy/colonoscopy Biopsy report	Type and screen for patients with Hg <10	Type and screen for patients in holding area with Hg <10	CBC
Interventions	Many or all of the above labs/diagnostics will have already been done. Check all results and fax to the surgeon's office.	Admit by 8 a.m. Check for bowel prep orders Bowel prep* Antiembolism stockings Incentive spirometry Ankle exercises* I.V. access* Routine VS* Pneumatic inflation boots	Shave and prep in O.R. Nasogastric(NG) tube maintenance* Intake and output (I/O) VS per routine* Foley care* Incentive spirometry* Ankle exercises* I.V. site care* Head of bed (HOB) 30° Safety measures* Wound care* Mouth care*	NG tube maintenance* I/O* VS per routine* Foley care* Incentive spirometry* Ankle exercises* I.V. site care* HOB 30°* Safety measures* Wound care* Mouth care* Antiembolism stockings
I.V.s		I.V.F.S., $D_5\frac{1}{2}$ NSS	I.V.F.S., D_5LR	I.V.F.S., LR
Medication	Prescribe GoLYTELY/Nulytely 10a—2p Neomycin @ 2p, 3p, and 10p Erythromycin @2p, 3p, and 10p	GoLYTELY/Nulytely 10a—2p Erythromycin @ 2p, 3p, and 10p Neomycin @ 2p, 3p and 10p	Preop ABX in holding area Postop ABX × 2 doses PCA (basal rate 0.5 mg) S.C. heparin	PCA (basal S.C. hepari
Diet/GI	Clears presurgery day NPO after midnight	Clears presurgery day NPO after midnight	NPO/NG tube	NPO/NG tube
Activity			4 hours after surgery ambulate with abdominal binder* D/C pneumatic inflation boots once patient ambulates	Ambulate t.i.d. with abdominal binder* May shower Physical therapy b.i.d.
KEY: *NSG Activities **V = Variance** **N = No Var.** **NSG care performed:** **Signatures:**	V V V N N N ☑ ☑ 1. _C. Malloy, RN_ 2. _____ 3. _____	V V V N N N ☑ ☑ 1. _M Connel, RN_ 2. _____ 3. _____	V V V N N N ☑ ☑ 1. _L. Singer, RN_ 2. _J. Smith, RN_ 3. _P. Joseph, RN_	V V V N N N ☑ ☑ 1. _L. Singer, RN_ 2. _J. Smith, RN_ 3. _P. Joseph, RN_

The pathway designates a specific time frame for patient care activities.

The pathway is organized into categories based on the patient's medical diagnosis.

The pathway lists tasks that the patient and caregivers need to accomplish.

(continued)

Take the critical pathway *(continued)*

CRITICAL PATHWAY: COLON RESECTION WITHOUT COLOSTOMY

	Postop Day 2	Postop Day 3	Postop Day 4	Postop Day 5
Assessments	Review of systems assessment*	Review of systems assessment*	Review of systems assessment*	Review of systems assessment*
Consults		Dietary consult		Oncology consult if indicated (Dukes B2 or C or high risk lesion) (or to be done as outpatient)
Labs and diagnostics	Electrolyte 7 (EL-7) Chest X-ray (CXR)	CBC EL-7	Pathology results on chart	CBC EL-7
Interventions	D/C NG tube if possible* (per guidelines) I/O* VS per routine* D/C Foley* ambulating* Incentive spirometry* Ankle exercises* I.V. site care* HOB 30°* Safety measures* Wound care* Mouth care* Antiembolism stockings	I/O* VS per routine* Incentive spirometry* Ankle exercises* I.V. site care* Safety measures* Wound care* Antiembolism stockings	I/O* VS per routine* Incentive spirometry* Ankle exercises* I.V. site care* Safety measures* Wound care* Antiembolism stockings	Consider staple removal Replace with Steri-Strips Assess that patient has met d/c criteria*
I.V.s	I.V.F.S D5½NSS+ MVI	I.V.-Heplock	Heplock	D/C Heplock
Medication	PCA (.5 mg basal rate)	D/C PCA P.O. analgesia Resume routine home meds	P.O. analgesia Preop meds	P.O. analgesia Preop meds
Diet/GI	D/C NG tube per guidelines: (Clamp tube at 8 a.m. if no N/V and residual <200 ml, D/C tube @ 12 noon)* (Check with doctor first)	Clears if+bm/flatus Advance to postop diet if tolerating clears (at least one tray of clears)*	House	House
Activity	Ambulate q.i.d. with abdominal binder* May shower Physical therapy b.i.d.	Ambulate at least q.i.d. with abdominal binder* May shower Physical therapy bid	Ambulate at least q.i.d. with abdominal binder* May shower Physical therapy b.i.d.	
Teaching	Reinforce preop teaching* Patient and family education p.r.n.* Re: family screening	Reinforce pre-op teaching* Patient and family education p.r.n.* Re: family screening begin D/C teaching	Reinforce preop teaching* Patient and family education p.r.n.* D/C teaching re: reportable s/s, F/U and wound care*	Review all D/C instructions and Rx including:* follow up appointments: with surgeon within 3 weeks with oncologist within 1 month if

The pathway lists key events that must occur before the patient's discharge date.

| **KEY: *NSG Activities** **V = Variance** **N = No Var.** **NSG care performed:** **Signatures:** | V V V ☑ ☑ ☑ 1. A. McCarthy, RN 2. R. Mayer, RN 3. | V V V ☑ ☑ ☑ 1. A. McCarthy, RN 2. R. Mayer, RN 3. | V V V ☑ ☑ ☑ 1. L. Singer, RN 2. J. Smith, RN 3. P. Joseph, RN | V V V ☑ ☑ ☑ 1. L. Singer, RN 2. J. Smith, RN 3. P. Joseph, RN |

There's always a drawback

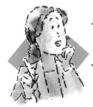

A significant disadvantage of critical pathways is that they're less effective for patients who have several diagnoses or who have complications. Establishing a time line for these patients is more difficult.

For example, treatment progress is usually predictable for a patient who has a cholecystectomy and is otherwise healthy. But if a patient has diabetes and coronary artery disease, the treatment course is fairly unpredictable, and the plan of care is likely to change. The result is lengthy and fragmented documentation.

A time for every purpose in the pathway

Just as you prioritize your nursing diagnoses, you must set priorities for the collaborative problems in the critical pathway. For example, if your patient needs whirlpool treatments by the physical therapy department and nebulizer treatments from a respiratory therapist, you must coordinate these activities according to the patient's current status and needs.

If everyone on the health care team plans carefully and pays attention to the patient's response to treatments, you should be able to carry out your respective activities for the patient's benefit.

Quick quiz

1. Before 1991, the nursing plan of care was:
   A. discarded when the patient was discharged.
   B. part of the patient's permanent record.
   C. used by doctors as well as nurses.

Answer: A. In 1991, JCAHO began requiring that the plan of care be permanently integrated into the patient's medical record.

2. People with access to the plan of care include:
   A. all caregivers, the patient, and members of his family.
   B. the nursing staff only.
   C. just nurses and doctors.

Answer: A. Besides caregivers, the patient and members of his family should use the plan of care and make recommendations and evaluations.

3. One way to get your patient to participate while he learns is:
  A. having him watch closed-circuit television.
  B. giving him medical textbooks to read (this may also help him sleep).
  C. return demonstration.

Answer: C. Patients can also participate in their learning through role playing and instructing other patients.

4. The three categories of learning behaviors and expected learning outcomes are:
  A. cognitive, psychomotor, and affective.
  B. cognizant, psychological, and effective.
  C. conscious, manual, and attitudinal.

Answer: A. Cognitive learning refers to understanding, psychomotor learning refers to manual skills, and affective learning refers to attitudes.

5. Compared to a standardized plan of care, a traditional plan is:
  A. easier to store on microfilm.
  B. easier to adapt to recent policy changes by the JCAHO.
  C. easier to tailor to the individual patient.

Answer: C. The traditional plan of care is written from scratch to meet the needs of an individual patient. Standardized plans are preprinted and based on interventions for patients with similar diagnoses.

Scoring

☆☆☆   If you answered all five items correctly, wow! You'll undoubtedly be nominated for a Pulitzer Prize for Outstanding Outcomes!

☆☆   If you answered three or four correctly, wonderful! Your plans are more than precise, they're poetic. You excel in traditional, standardized, and free-verse formats.

☆   If you answered fewer than three correctly, practice more planning! You'll soon win critical acclaim for your carefully crafted critical pathways!

Charting systems

In this chapter, you'll learn:

♦ about different types of charting systems and how to use them

♦ the advantages and disadvantages of various systems

♦ how to choose a charting system.

A look at charting systems

Different health care facilities set their own requirements for documentation and evaluation, but all must comply with legal, accreditation, and professional standards. A nursing department also may select a documentation system, as long as it adheres to those standards.

Narrative or alternative?

Depending on your facility's policy, you'll use one or more documentation systems to record your nursing interventions and evaluations and the patient's response. Some facilities use traditional narrative charting systems. Others choose alternative systems.

Each documentation system includes specific policies and procedures for charting, so make sure you understand the documentation requirements for the system your facility uses. Understanding and adhering to these requirements will help you to document care systematically and accurately. (See *Comparing charting systems,* page 56.)

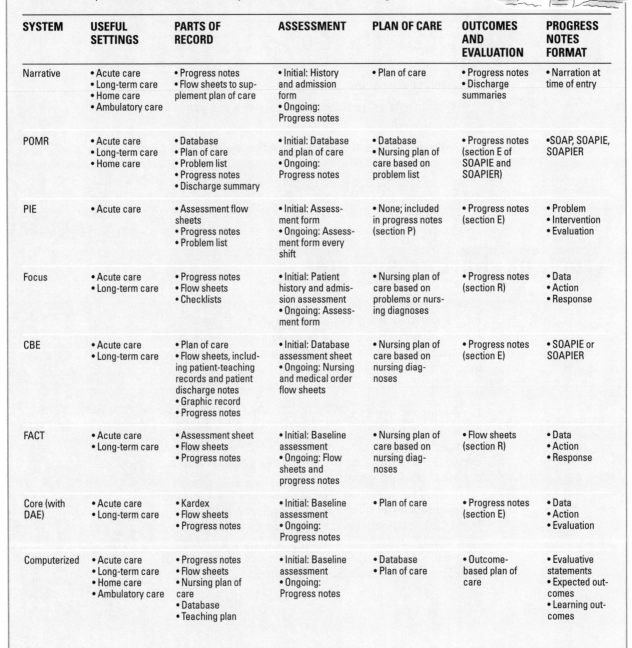

Comparing charting systems

The table below compares elements of the different charting systems used today. Note that the second column provides information on which systems work best in which settings.

SYSTEM	USEFUL SETTINGS	PARTS OF RECORD	ASSESSMENT	PLAN OF CARE	OUTCOMES AND EVALUATION	PROGRESS NOTES FORMAT
Narrative	• Acute care • Long-term care • Home care • Ambulatory care	• Progress notes • Flow sheets to supplement plan of care	• Initial: History and admission form • Ongoing: Progress notes	• Plan of care	• Progress notes • Discharge summaries	• Narration at time of entry
POMR	• Acute care • Long-term care • Home care	• Database • Plan of care • Problem list • Progress notes • Discharge summary	• Initial: Database and plan of care • Ongoing: Progress notes	• Database • Nursing plan of care based on problem list	• Progress notes (section E of SOAPIE and SOAPIER)	•SOAP, SOAPIE, SOAPIER
PIE	• Acute care	• Assessment flow sheets • Progress notes • Problem list	• Initial: Assessment form • Ongoing: Assessment form every shift	• None; included in progress notes (section P)	• Progress notes (section E)	• Problem • Intervention • Evaluation
Focus	• Acute care • Long-term care	• Progress notes • Flow sheets • Checklists	• Initial: Patient history and admission assessment • Ongoing: Assessment form	• Nursing plan of care based on problems or nursing diagnoses	• Progress notes (section R)	• Data • Action • Response
CBE	• Acute care • Long-term care	• Plan of care • Flow sheets, including patient-teaching records and patient discharge notes • Graphic record • Progress notes	• Initial: Database assessment sheet • Ongoing: Nursing and medical order flow sheets	• Nursing plan of care based on nursing diagnoses	• Progress notes (section E)	• SOAPIE or SOAPIER
FACT	• Acute care • Long-term care	• Assessment sheet • Flow sheets • Progress notes	• Initial: Baseline assessment • Ongoing: Flow sheets and progress notes	• Nursing plan of care based on nursing diagnoses	• Flow sheets (section R)	• Data • Action • Response
Core (with DAE)	• Acute care • Long-term care	• Kardex • Flow sheets • Progress notes	• Initial: Baseline assessment • Ongoing: Progress notes	• Plan of care	• Progress notes (section E)	• Data • Action • Evaluation
Computerized	• Acute care • Long-term care • Home care • Ambulatory care	• Progress notes • Flow sheets • Nursing plan of care • Database • Teaching plan	• Initial: Baseline assessment • Ongoing: Progress notes	• Database • Plan of care	• Outcome-based plan of care	• Evaluative statements • Expected outcomes • Learning outcomes

Traditional narrative

Narrative charting is a chronological account of:
• the patient's status
• the nursing interventions performed
• the patient's responses.

Today, few facilities rely on this system alone. Instead, they combine it with other systems, especially the source-oriented record.

Using narrative charting

In the traditional narrative system, the nurse usually records data as progress notes, with flow sheets supplementing the narrative notes. (See *Narrow in on narrative charting,* page 58.) Knowing when and what to document and how to organize the data are the key elements of effective narrative charting in the progress notes.

The Joint Commission on Accreditation of Healthcare Organizations (JCAHO) requires all health care facilities to establish policies on the frequency of patient reassessment. So assess your patient at least as often as required by your facility's policy, and then document your findings.

Documentation mania!

If you find yourself writing repetitious, meaningless notes, you may be documenting too often. If so, double-check your facility's policy. You may be following a time-consuming, unwritten standard initiated by staff members, not by your facility. To guard against this, review the policy at least every 6 months.

Observe and take note

Besides documenting when required by policy, be sure to write specific and descriptive narrative in the progress notes whenever you observe any of the following:
• a change in the patient's condition, such as progression, regression, or new problems. For example, write *The patient can ambulate with a walker for 3 minutes before feeling tired.*
• a patient's response to a treatment or medication. For example, write *The patient states that abdominal pain is relieved 1 hour after re-*

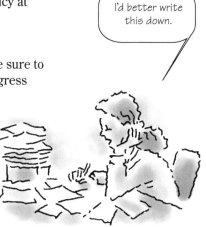

I'd better write this down.

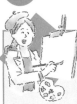

Art of the chart

Narrow in on narrative charting

This progress note is one example of narrative charting.

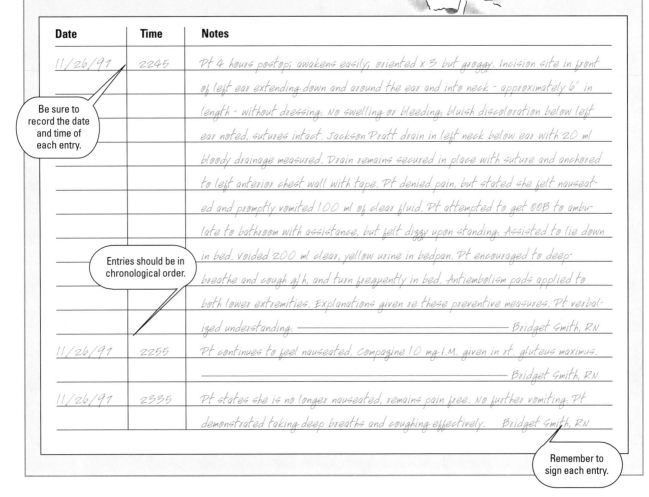

Date	Time	Notes
11/26/91	2245	Pt 4 hours postop; awakens easily; oriented x 3 but groggy. Incision site in front of left ear extending down and around the ear and into neck - approximately 6" in length - without dressing. No swelling or bleeding; bluish discoloration below left ear noted, sutures intact. Jackson Pratt drain in left neck below ear with 20 ml bloody drainage measured. Drain remains secured in place with suture and anchored to left anterior chest wall with tape. Pt denied pain, but stated she felt nauseated and promptly vomited 100 ml of clear fluid. Pt attempted to get OOB to ambulate to bathroom with assistance, but felt dizzy upon standing. Assisted to lie down in bed. Voided 200 ml clear, yellow urine in bedpan. Pt encouraged to deep-breathe and cough q/h, and turn frequently in bed. Antiembolism pads applied to both lower extremities. Explanations given re these preventive measures. Pt verbalized understanding. ———————————————— Bridget Smith, RN
11/26/91	2255	Pt continues to feel nauseated. Compazine 10 mg I.M. given in rt. gluteus maximus. ———————————————— Bridget Smith, RN
11/26/91	2335	Pt states she is no longer nauseated, remains pain free. No further vomiting. Pt demonstrated taking deep breaths and coughing effectively. Bridget Smith, RN

Be sure to record the date and time of each entry.

Entries should be in chronological order.

Remember to sign each entry.

ceiving medication. He's smiling and able to turn in bed without difficulty.

• a lack of improvement in the patient's condition. For example, write *No change in size or condition of sacral decubitus ulcer after 6 days of treatment. Dimensions and condition remain as stated in 11/20/97 note.*

• a patient's or family member's response to teaching. For example, write *The patient was able to demonstrate crutch-walking using the proper technique.*

One thought leads to another

Before you write anything, organize your thoughts so your paragraphs flow smoothly. If you have trouble deciding what to write, refer to the patient's plan of care to review the following:
• unresolved problems
• prescribed interventions
• expected outcomes.
Then write down your observations of the patient's progress in these areas. (See *Put your thoughts in order.*)

Advantages of narrative charting

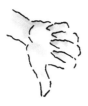

Narrative charting has a lot going for it. After all, this charting format:
• is the most flexible of all the charting systems, and is suitable in any clinical setting
• strongly conveys your nursing interventions and your patients' responses
• is ideal for presenting information that's collected over a long period
• combines well with other documentation devices, such as flow sheets, which cuts down on charting time
• uses narration, the most common form of writing, so training new staff members can usually be done quickly
• places its narrative notes in chronological order, so other team members can review the patient's progress on a day-to-day basis.

Disadvantages of narrative charting

On the other hand, narrative charting has some things working against it. They are:
• You have to read the entire record to find the patient outcome. Even then, you may have trouble determining the outcome of a problem because the same information may not be consistently documented.
• For the same reason, you may have trouble tracking problems and identifying trends in the patient's progress.
• Narrative charting offers no inherent guide to what's important to document, so nurses often document everything, resulting in a lengthy, repetitive record.

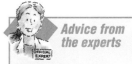
Advice from the experts

Put your thoughts in order

If you have trouble organizing your thoughts, use this sequence of questions to order your entry:
• How did I first become aware of the problem?
• What has the patient said about the problem that's significant?
• What have I observed that's related to the problem?
• What is my plan for dealing with the problem?
• What steps have I taken to intervene?
• How has the patient responded to my interventions?

To make your notes as coherent as possible, discuss each of the patient's problems in a separate paragraph; don't lump them together. Or, use a head-to-toe approach to organize your information.

Be sure to notify the doctor of significant changes that you observe. Then document this communication, the doctor's responses, and any new orders to be implemented.

• Narratives may contain vague or inaccurate language, such as "appears to be bleeding" or "small amount."

You may be able to avoid some disadvantages of narrative charting by organizing the information you record. (See *AIR: A fresh narrative format*.)

Problem-oriented medical record

The problem-oriented medical record (POMR) focuses on specific patient problems. It was originally developed by doctors and later adapted by nurses. The POMR is most effective in acute care or long-term care settings.

AIR: A fresh narrative format

A charting format called AIR may help you to organize and simplify your narrative charting. AIR is an acronym for:
• **A**ssessment
• **I**ntervention
• **R**esponse.

The AIR format synthesizes major nursing events while avoiding repetition of information found elsewhere in the medical record. Combined with nursing flow sheets and the nursing plan of care, the AIR format can be used to document the care you provide clearly and concisely.

Here's how AIR is used to document nursing care.

Assessment
Summarize your physical assessment findings. Begin by specifying each issue that you address, such as nursing diagnosis, admission note, and discharge planning. Rather than simply describing the patient's current condition, document trends and record your impression of the problem.

Intervention
Summarize your actions and those of other caregivers in response to the assessment data. The summary may include a condensed nursing plan of care or plans for additional patient monitoring.

Response
Summarize the outcome or the patient's response to the nursing interventions. Because a response may not be evident for hours or even days, this documentation may not immediately follow the entries. In fact, it may be recorded by another nurse, which is why titling each of your assessments and interventions is so important.

Multidisciplinary mania!

In this charting system, you describe each problem in multidisciplinary patient progress notes (not on progress notes with only nursing information).

Five-part format

The POMR is divided into five parts:

☝ database

✌ problem list

🖐 initial plan

✋ progress notes

🖖 discharge summary.

In POMR charting, you record your interventions and evaluations in the progress notes and discharge summary only. But to really understand POMR, review all five parts.

Database

Usually completed by a nurse, the database, or initial assessment, is the foundation for the patient's plan of care. A collection of subjective and objective information about the patient, the database includes the reason for hospitalization, medical history, allergies, medication regimen, physical and psychosocial findings, self-care abilities, educational needs, and other discharge planning concerns. The database is the basis for a problem list.

Problem list

After analyzing the database, various caregivers list the patient's current problems in chronological order according to the date when each is identified (not in order of acuteness or priority). This list provides an overview of the patient's health status.

Originally, POMR called for one interdisciplinary problem list. Although this may still be done, nurses and doctors usually keep separate lists with problems stated as either nursing or medical diagnoses.

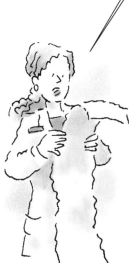

My database forms the basis for a problem list.

Number 'em

As you list the patient's problems, number them so they correspond to the problems in the rest of the POMR. Have every entry on the patient's initial plan, progress notes, and discharge summary correspond to a number. File the numbered problem list at the front of the patient's chart. Keep the list current by adding new numbers as new problems arise. When writing notes, be sure to identify the problem you're discussing by the appropriate number.

No longer a problem

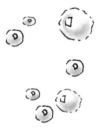

Once you've resolved a problem, draw a line through it. Or show that it's inactive by retiring the problem number and highlighting the problem with a colored felt-tip pen. Don't use that number again for the same patient.

Initial plan

After constructing the problem list, write an initial plan for each problem. This plan includes:
• expected outcomes
• plans for further data collection, if needed
• patient care
• teaching plans.
    Involve the patient in goal setting as you construct the initial plan. This fosters the patient's compliance and is essential to the effectiveness of your interventions.

Progress notes

One of the most prominent features of the POMR is the structured way that narrative progress notes are written by all team members using the SOAP, SOAPIE, or SOAPIER format. (See *SOAP, SOAPIE, SOAPIER charting.*)
    Usually, you must write a complete note in one of these formats every 24 hours whenever a problem is unresolved or the patient's condition changes.
    You don't need to write an entry for each SOAP or SOAPIE component every time you document. If you have nothing to record for a component, either omit the letter from the note or leave a blank space after it, depending on your facility's policy. (See *Problem-oriented progress notes,* page 65.)

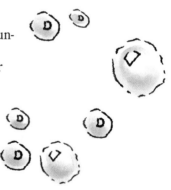

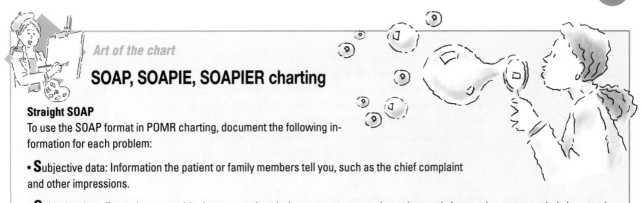

Art of the chart

SOAP, SOAPIE, SOAPIER charting

Straight SOAP

To use the SOAP format in POMR charting, document the following information for each problem:

• **S**ubjective data: Information the patient or family members tell you, such as the chief complaint and other impressions.

• **O**bjective data: Factual, measurable data you gather during assessment, such as observed signs and symptoms, vital signs, and laboratory test values.

• **A**ssessment data: Conclusions based on the collected subjective and objective data and formulated as patient problems or nursing diagnoses. This dynamic and ongoing process changes as more or different subjective and objective information becomes known.

• **P**lan: Your strategy for relieving the patient's problem. This plan should include both immediate or short-term actions and long-term measures.

It's getting SOAPIE

Some facilities use the SOAPIE format, adding the following to SOAP:

• **I**ntervention: Measures you take to achieve an expected outcome. As the patient's health status changes, you may need to modify your interventions. Be sure to document the patient's understanding and acceptance of the initial plan in this section of your notes.

• **E**valuation: An analysis of the effectiveness of your interventions.

It's even SOAPIER

The SOAPIER format adds a revision section for the documentation of alternative interventions. If your patient's outcomes fall short of expectations, use the evaluation process called for in SOAPIE as a basis for developing revised interventions, then document these changes:

• **R**evision: Document any changes from the original plan of care in this section. Interventions, outcomes, or target dates may need to be adjusted to reach a previous goal.

Discharge summary

The discharge summary — the last part of POMR — covers each problem on the list and notes whether it was resolved. This is the place in your SOAP or SOAPIE note to discuss any unresolved problems and to outline your plan for dealing with the problem after discharge. Also record communications with other facilities, home health agencies, and the patient.

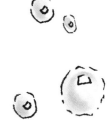

Pros of the POMR

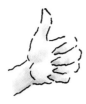

The POMR charting system has several advantages:
• Information about each problem is organized into specific categories that all caregivers can understand. This eases data retrieval and communication between disciplines.
• Continuity of care is shown by combining the plan of care and progress notes into a complete record of the care that's planned and care that's delivered. The caregiver addresses each problem or nursing diagnosis in the nurses' notes.
• It encourages nurses to document the nursing process, to chart more consistently, and to chart only essential data.

Cons of the POMR

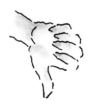

The POMR system also has some disadvantages. For example:
• The emphasis on the chronology of problems, rather than their priority, may cause caregivers to disagree about which problems to list.
• Trends may be hard to analyze if information is buried in the daily narrative.
• Both assessments and interventions apply to more than one problem, so charting of these findings is repetitious, especially with the SOAPIE format. This makes documentation time-consuming to perform and to read.
• The format emphasizes problems, so routine care may be left undocumented unless flow sheets are used.
• The format doesn't work well in settings with rapid patient turnover, such as a postanesthesia care unit, short procedure unit, or emergency department.
• Problems may arise if caregivers don't keep the problem list current or if they're confused about which problems to list.
• Considerable time and cost are needed to train people to use the SOAP, SOAPIE, and SOAPIER method.

Problem-intervention-evaluation

The problem-intervention-evaluation (PIE) system organizes information according to patients' problems and was devised to simplify the documentation process.

This system requires you to keep a daily patient assessment flow sheet and progress notes. Integrating the

Art of the chart

Problem-oriented progress notes

The table below is an example of progress notes as they appear in a problem-oriented medical record.

No problem!

Number each problem for easy reference.

Progress notes are in SOAPIE format.

Date	Time	Notes
11/1/91	0645	#1 Pain
		S: Pt states "I am having severe back pain again."
		O: Pt states pain is #9 on 1 to 10 scale; skin is warm, pale, moist. Pt is restless, pacing in room, holding right flank area with his hand; pt also complaining of nausea.
		A: Pt in severe pain, needs medication for relief.
		P: Check orders for analgesia; check for any allergies; take V.S.; if within normal limits, give analgesia as ordered. Recheck pt in 30 minutes for response. Monitor pt for adverse reactions to drug. Observe pt for pain frequently; offer medication as ordered before pain becomes severe. ———————— Ann Davis, RN
11/1/91	0651	#1 Pain
		S: Pt states "The pain is less."
		O: Pt states his pain is now a #2 on 1 to 10 scale. Skin warm, dry, color normal. Pt sitting on bed, watching the news. No further nausea.
		A: Pt is improved.
		P: Continue to monitor for pain and other symptoms.
		I: BP 158/84, pulse 104, RR 24 - meperidine 75 mg and hydroxyzine 50 mg I.M., left gluteus maximus.
		E: Medication was effective. ———————— Ann Davis, RN
11/1/91	0130	#2 Anxiety
		S: Pt states "I am worried about the surgery and being out of work."
		O: Pt wringing his hands, eyes downcast.
		A: Pt is anxious regarding upcoming surgery and its impact on his job.
		P: Encourage verbalization of feelings and concerns. Offer emotional support. Involve family to discuss his concerns if agreeable to pt. ———————— Ann Davis, RN
11/1/91	0130	#3 Risk for postop surgical complications
		S: Pt states "I never had surgery before."
		O: Pt is unsure about what to expect.
		A: Pt needs preop and postop education.
		P: Teach pt about events before and after surgery; for example, I.V. insertion; teach about the need for coughing and deep breathing; moving frequently in bed, and early ambulation after surgery. Explain why these are important. Evaluate pt's response to the teaching and document. ———————— Ann Davis, RN

plan of care into the nurses' progress notes eliminates the need for a separate plan of care. The idea is to provide a concise, efficient record of patient care that has a nursing focus. (See *Easy as PIE*.)

Using the PIE system

To use the PIE system, first assess the patient and document your findings on a daily patient assessment flow sheet.

Pieces of PIE

The daily assessment flow sheet lists defined assessment terms under major categories, such as respiration, along with routine care and monitoring measures, such as providing ventilation and monitoring breath sounds. The flow sheet generally includes space to record pertinent treatments.

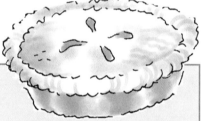

Art of the chart

Easy as PIE

This sample chart shows how to write progress notes using the problem-intervention-evaluation (PIE) system.

Date	Time	Notes
12/20/91	1300	P#1: Sudden onset of generalized itching and hives possibly related to an allergic reaction.
		IP#1: Note extent of symptoms; take vital signs; assess breath sounds for wheezing. Notify doctor immediately. Administer medications as ordered, including I.V. access. Reassure pt.
		EP#1: Symptoms abate; pt maintains adequate respiratory and hemodynamic status; pt verbalized understanding of treatments and need to report further symptoms. ———— Mary Smith, RN
12/20/91	1300	P#2: High risk for ineffective breathing pattern related to possible allergic reaction.
		IP#2: Take vital signs frequently and monitor breath sounds and pulse oximetry. Notify doctor for abnormal pulse oximetry or wheezing. Give meds as ordered. Teach pt signs of respiratory distress and the need to report these immediately. ———— Mary Smith, RN
		EP#2: Pt will have no wheezing or dyspnea; pt verbalized understanding of need to notify nurse of changes in breathing patterns. ———— Mary Smith, RN

This stands for evaluation of problem number 1.

After a problem is resolved, draw a line through it to indicate that it's no longer current.

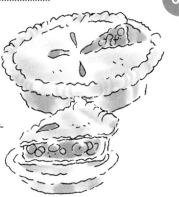

On the flow sheet, initial only the assessment terms that apply to your patient and mark abnormal findings with an asterisk. Record detailed information in your progress notes.

Next, chart the patient's problems, your interventions, and your evaluations of the patient's responses.

Problem

After performing and documenting an initial assessment, use the collected data to identify pertinent nursing diagnoses. These form the *problem* piece of PIE. Use the list of nursing diagnoses accepted by your facility, which usually corresponds to the diagnoses approved by the North American Nursing Diagnosis Association (NANDA).

Got a problem with that?

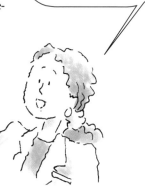

Number each problem for future reference.

If you can't find a nursing diagnosis on an approved list, write the problem statement yourself using accepted criteria.

In the progress notes, document all nursing diagnoses or problems, labeling each as *P* and numbering it. For example, the first nursing diagnosis is labeled *P #1*. This way, you can later refer to a specific problem by its label only, without having to redocument the problem statement. Some facilities also use a separate problem-list form to keep a convenient running account of the nursing diagnoses for each patient.

Intervention

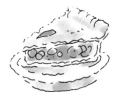

To chart the *intervention* piece of PIE, document the nursing actions you take for each nursing diagnosis. Write them on the progress sheet, labeling each as *I* and assigning the appropriate problem number. For example, to refer to an intervention for the first nursing diagnosis, write *IP #1*.

Evaluation

After charting your interventions, document the patient's responses in your progress notes. These form the *evaluation* piece of PIE. Use the label *E* followed by the assigned problem number. For example, to identify each evaluation write *EP #1*.

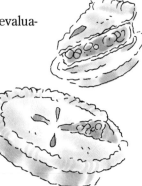

Reevaluate and review

Make sure that you or another nurse evaluates each problem at least once every 8 hours. After every three shifts, review the notes from the previous 24 hours to identify the patient's current problems and responses to interventions.

Document continuing problems daily, along with relevant interventions and evaluations. Cross out resolved problems from the daily documentation.

Pros of PIE

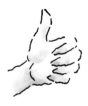

The PIE format has many attractive features, including:
• ensuring that your documentation includes all the necessary pieces: nursing diagnoses (problems), related interventions, and evaluations
• encouraging you to meet JCAHO requirements by providing an organized framework for your thoughts and writing
• simplifying documentation by combining the plan of care and progress notes
• improving the quality of your progress notes by highlighting interventions and requiring a written evaluation of the patient's response to them.

Cons of PIE

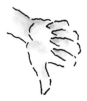

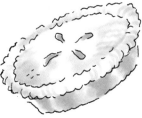

Don't take a "pie-in-the-sky" attitude to this charting system. Here's why:
• Staff members may need in-depth training before they can use it.
• It requires you to re-evaluate each problem once every shift, which is time-consuming, often unnecessary, and leads to repetitive entries.
• It omits documentation of the planning step in the nursing process. This step, which addresses expected outcomes, is essential in evaluating the patient's responses.
• It doesn't incorporate multidisciplinary charting.

Focus system

Nurses who found the SOAP format awkward developed the focus system of charting. This system is organized into patient-centered topics, or *foci*. It encourages you to use assessment data to evaluate these concerns. Focus charting works best in acute care settings and on units where the same care and procedures are repeated frequently.

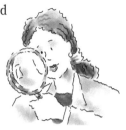

Coming into focus

To implement focus documentation, you use a progress sheet with columns for the date, time, focus, and progress notes. (See *Focus on focus charting,* page 70.) You can identify the foci by reviewing your assessment data.

In focus charting, you typically write each focus as a nursing diagnosis, such as *risk for infection* or *fluid volume deficit.* However, the focus also may refer to the following:

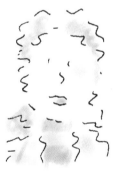
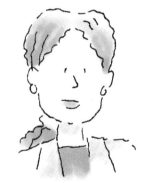

- a sign or symptom, such as purulent drainage or chest pain
- a patient behavior such as inability to ambulate
- a special need such as a discharge need
- an acute change in the patient's condition, such as loss of consciousness or increase in blood pressure
- a significant event such as surgery.

Writing focus progress notes

In the progress notes column, divide the information into three categories: data (D), action (A), and response (R).

In the data category, include subjective and objective information that describes the focus.

In the action category, include immediate and future nursing actions based on your assessment of the patient's

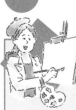

Art of the chart

Focus on focus charting

The table below is an example of progress notes when using the focus system.

> Progress notes are divided into data, action, and response.

> This focus is written as a nursing diagnosis.

Date	Time	Focus	Progress notes
8/3/91	1000	Knowledge deficit R/T diagnosis	D: Pt states she does not understand what her diagnosis means.
			A: Illness explained to pt according to her level of understanding. Pt taught symptoms she may expect and why she is having current symptoms. Treatments and procedures explained. Questions answered. Pt encouraged to verbalize need for further instruction or information.
			R: Pt verbalized better understanding of her illness.————————— Donna Jones, RN
8/3/91	1000	Abnormal vaginal bleeding	D: Pt states her period just began and she is passing a large amount of clots.
			A: Amount of bleeding assessed. Pt saturated 2 maxi pads in the past hour, currently large amount of bright red clots noted. BP 114/70 HR 98 RR 20. Pt status reported to doctor. Orders received. 20G I.V. catheter started, labs drawn; 1,000 ml NSS hung; macro tubing, at 100 ml/hr. Pt tolerated procedures well. Will continue to monitor vital signs and bleeding. Dr. Smith will be in to see pt. Pt taught how to assess amount of vaginal drainage.
			R: Pt verbalizes correct amount of drainage and type. Pt understands procedures. Donna Jones, RN
8/3/91	1000	Anxiety	D: Pt states "I'm afraid of all this blood."
			A: Emotional support provided. Encouraged verbalization. Explanations given regarding treatments and procedures. Family in to provide support.
			R: Pt observed talking and laughing with family. States she feels less anxious. Donna Jones, RN

> The focus zooms in on the topics of major concern.

condition. This category also includes changes to the plan of care as necessary, based on your evaluation.

In the response category, describe the patient's response to nursing or medical care.

Lights, camera, data, action, response!

Using all three categories guarantees complete documentation based on the nursing process. Be sure to record routine nursing tasks and assessment data on your flow sheets and checklists.

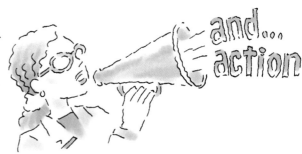

Advantages of focus charting

Focus charting has several strong points. For example:
• It's flexible enough to adapt to any clinical setting.
• It centers on the nursing process, and the data-action-response format encourages you to record in a process-oriented way.
• Information on a specific problem is easy to find because the focus statement is separate from the progress note. This also promotes communication between health care team members.
• It encourages regular documentation of patient responses to nursing and medical care and ensures adherence to JCAHO requirements.
• You can use this format to document many topics besides those on the problem list or plan of care.
• It helps you organize your thoughts and document succinctly and precisely.
• It helps you identify areas in the plan of care that need revising as you document each entry.

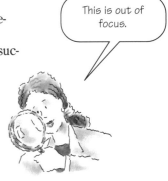

This is out of focus.

Disadvantages of focus charting

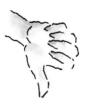

Focus charting also has weaknesses. For example:
• Staff members — especially those who are used to other systems — may need in-depth training before they can use it.
• You need to use many flow sheets and checklists, which can cause inconsistent documentation and problems tracking a patient's problems.
• If you forget to include the patient's response to interventions, focus charting resembles a long narrative, like that seen in progress notes.

Charting by exception

The system called charting by exception (CBE) was designed to eliminate lengthy and repetitive notes, poorly organized information, difficult-to-retrieve data, errors of omission, and other long-standing charting problems.

To avoid these pitfalls, the CBE format radically departs from traditional systems by requiring documentation of significant or abnormal findings only.

CBE guidelines

To use CBE effectively, you must adhere to established guidelines for nursing assessments and interventions and follow written standards of practice that identify the nurse's basic responsibilities.

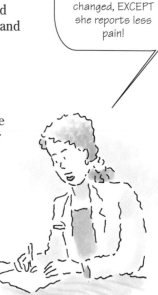

This patient's condition is unchanged, EXCEPT she reports less pain!

Document deviations

Guidelines for each body system are printed on CBE forms. For example, care standards for patient hygiene might specify a complete linen change every 3 days or sooner, if necessary. Having the standards clearly and concisely written eliminates the need to chart routine nursing care or any other care outlined in the standards. All you document are deviations from the standards.

Get your guidelines here

Guidelines for interventions used in the CBE system come from these sources:
- *nursing diagnosis–based standardized plans of care.* These identify patient problems, desired outcomes, and interventions.
- *patient care guidelines.* These are standardized interventions created for specific patients such as those with a nursing diagnosis of pain. These guidelines outline the nursing interventions, treatments, and time frame for repeated assessments.
- *doctor's orders.* These are prescribed medical interventions.
- *incidental orders.* These are usually one-time, miscellaneous nursing or medical orders or interdependent interventions related to a protocol or a piece of equipment.
- *standards of nursing practice.* These define the acceptable level of routine nursing care for all patients. They may describe the essential aspects of nursing practice for a specific unit or for all clinical areas.

CBE format

The CBE format includes a standardized plan of care based on the nursing diagnosis and several types of flow sheets. These flow sheets include:
- nursing and medical order flow sheet
- graphic form

• patient-teaching record
• patient discharge note.
    Sometimes, you may need to supplement your CBE documentation by using nurses' progress notes.

Standardized plans of care

When using the CBE format for charting, you fill out a preprinted plan of care for each nursing diagnosis.

Fill in the blanks

The preprinted plans of care have blank spaces so you can individualize them as needed. For example, include expected outcomes and major revisions in your plan of care. Place the completed forms in the nurses' progress notes section of the clinical record.

Nursing and medical order flow sheets

Use nursing and medical order flow sheets to document your assessments and interventions. Each flow sheet covers a 24-hour period of care for one patient.
    The top part of the flow sheet contains the doctor's orders for assessments and interventions. Each nursing order includes a corresponding nursing diagnosis, labeled *ND 1, ND 2,* and so on; doctor's orders are labeled *DO.* (See *Using a nursing and medical order flow sheet,* page 74.)

Checks, asterisks, and arrows

In addition to the abbreviations, ND for nursing diagnosis and DO for doctor's orders, use these symbols when you record care on flow sheets:
• a check mark (✔) to indicate a completed medical order or nursing assessment with no abnormal findings
• an asterisk (✱) to indicate an abnormal finding on an assessment or an abnormal response to an intervention
• an arrow (➔) to indicate that the patient's status hasn't changed since the previous entry.
    After completing an assessment, compare your findings with the printed guidelines on the back of the form. If a finding is within normal parameters, place a check mark in the appropriate box. If a finding isn't within the normal range, put an asterisk in the box. Then explain your findings in the comments section on the form.

Art of the chart

Using a nursing and medical order flow sheet

Here are the typical features of a nursing and medical order flow sheet.

> Asterisk indicates an abnormal assessment finding.

NURSING AND MEDICAL ORDER FLOW SHEET

Date 1/22/91

ND #/DO	Assessments and interventions		
ND 1	Wound assessment	0100*	1500*
ND 2	Range of motion assessment		
DO	Ancef 2g I.V. stat x 1/1 dose	0645✔	
Initials		CF	CF

Key
- DO = doctor's orders
- ND = nursing diagnosis
- ✔ = normal findings

- → = no change in condition
- ✳ = abnormal or significant finding (see Comments section)

ND #/DO	Time	Comments	Initials
ND 1	0800	Right leg wound with yellow drainage, inflammation around border. Doctor notified. No complaint of pain.	CF
ND 1	0830	Pt able to move both lower extremities 1" off bed.	CF
ND 1	1100	No drainage on R leg dressing	CF
ND 2	1100	Pt rates pain decreased to a 3.	CF
Initials CF		**Signature** Cary Filiaano, RN	

> Explain your findings in the comments section.

Note normalcy

An assessment finding that's not defined in the guidelines may be normal for a particular patient. For example, unclear speech may be normal in a patient with a long-standing tracheostomy. Reference this type of note by nursing diagnosis number or doctor's order and time. If the patient's condition hasn't changed from the last assessment, draw a horizontal arrow from the previous category box to the current one.

Make more marks

Document interventions similarly. Use a check mark to indicate a completed intervention and an expected patient response. Indicate significant findings or abnormal patient responses with an asterisk, and write an explanation in the comments section. When the patient's response is unchanged, use an arrow.

After you document an entire column in the assessments and interventions section, initial it at the bottom. Also initial all your entries in the comments section, and sign the form at the bottom of the page.

> Check for normal, asterisk for abnormal.

Care-full combinations

Some facilities use a special nursing care flow sheet that combines all the necessary forms, such as the graphic record, the daily activities checklist, and the patient care assessment section. (See *It flows together: Using a combined nursing care flow sheet,* pages 76 to 78.)

Graphic form

This section of a flow sheet is used to document trends in the patient's vital signs, weight, intake and output, and stool, urination, appetite, and activity levels.

More checks and asterisks

As with the nursing and medical order flow sheet, use check marks to indicate expected findings and asterisks to indicate abnormal ones. Record information about abnormalities in the nurses' progress notes or on the nursing and medical order flow sheet.

In the box labeled "routine standards," check off the established nursing care interventions you performed such as providing hygiene. Don't rewrite these standards as orders on the nursing and medical order flow sheet. Refer to the guidelines on the back of the graphic form for complete instructions.

Patient-teaching record

Use the patient-teaching form (or section) to identify the information, psychomotor skills, and social or behavioral measures that your patient or his caregiver must learn by a predetermined date. This record includes teaching resources, dates of patient achievements, and other pertinent observations. If the patient has multiple learning needs, you can use more than one form.

(Text continues on page 79.)

Art of the chart

It flows together: Using a combined nursing care flow sheet

This sample shows a portion of a nursing care flow sheet that combines a graphic record, a daily nursing care activities checklist, and a patient care assessment form.

> The graphic record makes it easy to spot trends.

Name _Maureen Gollen_

Date		12/29/91											
Hour		0700	0800	0900	1000	1100	1200	1300	1400	1500	1600	1700	1800
Temperature													

°C	°F
40.4	105
40.0	104
39.4	103
38.9	102
37.8	100
37.2	99
36.7	98
36.1	97
35.6	96

		0700	0800	0900	1000	1100	1200	1300	1400	1500	1600	1700	1800
Pulse		84	80	82	78	76	78	78	82	84	82	80	78
Respiration		16	20	20	22	24	24	18	20	22	20	18	24
BP	Lying												
	Sitting	136/82	130/80	126/74	132/82	132/80	140/82	136/74	130/70	138/78	140/80	132/78	136/76
	Standing												
Intake	Oral	240					360						120
	Tube												
	I.V.												
	Blood												
8-Hour total		600											
Output		400					450						
Other													
8-Hour total		850											
Teaching		dressing changes, s/s of infection											
Signature		Mary Murphy, RN								Ann Burns, RN			
		0700 - 1500								1500 - 2300			

It flows together: Using a combined nursing care flow sheet *(continued)*

This section allows for efficient documentation of daily activities.

	Hour	0700	0800	0900	1000	1100	1200	1300	1400	1500	1600	1700
ACTIVITY	Bed rest	MM							→	AB —		→
	OOB											
	Ambulate (assist)											
	Ambulatory											
	Sleeping											
	Bathroom privileges											
	HOB elevated	MM							→	AB —		→
	Cough, deep-breathe, turn		MM								AB	
	ROM Active / Passive		MM								AB	
HYGIENE	Bath		MM									
	Shave		MM									
	Oral		MM									
	Skin care											
	Peri care											
NUTRITION	Diet	House										
	% Eating			75%			60%					75%
	Feeding											
	Supplemental											
	S-Self, A-Assist, F-Feed		A				A					A
BLADDER	Catheter	indwelling urinary #18 Fr.										
	Incontinent											
	Voiding	clear, yellow urine										
	Intermittent catheter											
BOWEL	Stools (occult blood + or -)											
	Incontinent											
	Normal	large formed brown stool										
	Enema											
SPECIAL TREATMENTS	Special mattress	Low-pressure airflow mattress applied 0900										
	Special bed											
	Heel and elbow pads											
	Antiembolism stockings											
	Traction: + = on, - = off											
	Isolation type											

(continued)

It flows together: Using a combined nursing care flow sheet (continued)

ASSESSMENT FINDINGS

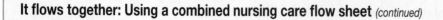

Findings marked by an asterisk need to be documented.

KEY: ✔ = normal findings
     ✳ = significant findings

	Day	Evening	Night	
Neurologic	✳ MM	✔ AB		0800 Limited ROM ® shoulder. Pt. states, "I have arthritis and my shoulder is always stiff."
Cardiovascular(CV)	✔ MM	✔ AB		
Respiratory	✔ MM	✳ AB		1800 Shallow breathing with poor inspiratory effort at 1700.
GI	✔ MM	✔ AB		
Genitourinary (GU)	✔ MM	✔ AB		
Surgical dressing and incision	✳ MM	✔ AB		0930 Incision reddened; dime-sized area of serous sanguineous drainage on old dressing
Skin integrity	✔ MM	✔ AB		
Psychosocial	✔ MM	✔ AB		
Educational	✳ MM	✔ AB		0945 Taught pt incisional care and dressing change, and s/s of infection
Peripheral vascular	✔ MM	✔ AB		

NORMAL ASSESSMENT FINDINGS

Neurologic assessment:
- Alert and oriented to person, place, and time.
- Speech clear and understandable.
- Memory intact.
- Behavior appropriate to situation and accommodation.
- Active range of motion (ROM) of all extremities, symmetrically equal strength.
- No paresthesia.

Cardiovascular assessment:
- Regular apical pulse.
- Palpable bilateral peripheral pulses.
- No peripheral edema.
- No calf tenderness.

Pulmonary assessment:
- Resting respirations 10 to 20 per minute, quiet and regular.
- Clear sputum.
- Pink nailbeds and mucous membranes.

Gastrointestinal assessment:
- Abdomen soft and nondistended.
- Tolerates prescribed diet without nausea or vomiting.
- Bowel movements within own normal pattern and consistency (as described in Patient Profile).

Genitourinary assessment:
- No indwelling catheter in use.
- Urinates without pain.
- Undistended bladder after urination.
- Urine is clear, yellow to amber color.

Surgical dressing and incision assessment:
- Dressing dry and intact.
- No evidence of redness, increased temperature, or tenderness in surrounding tissue.
- Sutures, staples, or Steri-Strips intact.
- Wound edges well-approximated.
- No drainage present.

Skin integrity assessment:
- Skin color normal.
- Skin warm, dry, and intact.
- Moist mucous membranes.

Psychosocial assessment:
- Interacts and communicates in an appropriate manner with others (family, significant others, health care personnel).

Educational assessment:
- Patient or significant others communicate understanding of the patient's health status, plan of care, and expected response.
- Patient or significant others demonstrate ability to perform health-related procedures and behaviors as taught.
- Items taught and expected performance must be specifically described in Significant Findings Section.

Peripheral vascular assessment:
- Affected extremity is pink, warm, and movable within average ROM.
- Capillary refill time less than 3 seconds.
- Peripheral pulses palpable.
- No edema, sensation intact without numbness or paresthesia.
- No pain on passive stretch.

Patient discharge note

Like other discharge forms, the patient discharge note is a flow sheet for documenting ongoing discharge planning. To chart discharge planning, follow the instructions printed on the back of the form. A typical discharge note includes patient instructions, appointments for follow-up care, medication and diet instructions, signs and symptoms to report, level of activity, and patient education.

Progress notes

Use the progress notes to document revisions in the plan of care and interventions that don't lend themselves to the nursing and medical order flow sheet. Because the CBE format allows you to document most assessments and interventions on the nursing and medical order flow sheet, your progress notes usually contain little assessment and intervention data.

Advantages of CBE

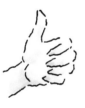

The CBE format has several important benefits:
• It eliminates documentation of routine care through the use of nursing care standards. This stops redundancies and clearly identifies abnormal data.
• Information that has already been recorded isn't repeated. For instance, you don't have to write a long entry each time you assess a patient if his condition stays the same.
• The use of well-defined guidelines and standards of care promotes uniform nursing practice.
• The flow sheets let you track trends easily.
• Guidelines are printed on the forms for ready reference. Abnormal findings are highlighted to help you quickly pinpoint significant changes and trends in a patient's condition.
• Patient data are immediately written on the permanent record. Because you don't need to keep temporary notes and then transcribe them onto the patient's chart later, all caregivers always have access to the most current data.
• Assessments are standardized so all caregivers evaluate and document findings consistently.

With CBE, I don't waste time charting routine care.

• All flow sheets are kept at the patient's bedside, where they serve as a ready reference. This encourages immediate documentation.

Disadvantages of CBE

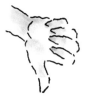

Nothing's perfect, including the CBE system. Here are the drawbacks:

• The development of clear guidelines and standards of care is time-consuming. For legal reasons, these guidelines and standards must be written and understood by all nurses before the system can be implemented.

• This system takes a long time for people to learn, accept, and use correctly and consistently.

• Narrative notes and evaluations of patients' responses may be brief and sketchy in facilities that use multiple forms instead of one combination form.

• This system was developed for RNs. Before LPNs can use it, it must be evaluated and modified to meet their scope of practice.

• This system, although legally sound, may be questioned in court until it becomes more widely known.

FACT documentation system

The computer-ready FACT documentation system incorporates many CBE principles. It was developed to help caregivers avoid the documentation of irrelevant data, repetitive notes, and inconsistencies among departments, and to reduce the amount of time spent charting.

Using the FACT system

In this system, you document only exceptions to the norm or significant information about the patient. The format uses an assessment and action flow sheet, a frequent assessment flow sheet, and progress notes. The content of flow sheets and notes may be individualized to some extent. The flow sheets cover a 24- to 72-hour time span, and you'll need to date, time, and sign all entries. (See *Face facts with FACT charting*.)

Memory Jogger

"FACT" is an acronym for the four key elements of this charting system. Here's how to remember these elements:

Flow sheets individualized to specific services

Assessment features standardized with baseline parameters

Concise, integrated progress notes and flow sheets documenting the patient's condition and responses

Timely entries recorded when care is given.

This system eliminates repetitive charting.

▶ *Art of the chart*

Face facts with FACT charting

This sample shows portions of an assessment flow sheet and a postoperative flow sheet using the FACT format.

Assessment parameters for each body system are on the form.

ASSESSMENT RECORD

	Date Time	12/18/91 0100	12/18/91 0500	12/18/91 0900
Neurologic Alert and oriented to time, place, and person. PERLA. Symmetry of strength in extremities. No difficulty with coordination. Behavior appropriate to situation. Sensation intact without numbness or paresthesia.		✓		✓
Orient patient.				
Refer to neurologic flow sheet.				
Pain No report of pain. If present, include patient statements about intensity (0 to 5 scale), location, description, duration, radiation, precipitating and alleviating factors.		5 - Neck pain	✓	1- Neck pain "It hurts."
Location		Cervical spine area		Cervical spine area
Relief measures		Pt repositioned		Percocet † p.o.
Pain relief: Yes/No		Y		Y
Cardiac Apical pulse 60 to 100. S_1 and S_2 present. Regular rhythm. Peripheral (radial, pedal) pulses present. No edema or calf tenderness. Extremities pink, warm, movable within patient's ROM.		✓	✓	✓
I.V. solution and rate		D_5 ½ NSS @ KVO	D_5 ½ NSS @ KVO	D_5 ½ NSS @ KVO
Pulmonary Respiratory rate 12 to 20 at rest, quiet, regular and nonlabored. Lungs clear and aerated equally in all lobes. No SOB at rest. No abnormal lung sounds. Mucous membranes pink.		✓	✓	✓
O_2 therapy				
Taught coughing, deep breathing, incentive spirometer		✓	✓	✓
Musculoskeletal Extremities pink, warm, and without edema; sensation and motion present. Normal joint ROM, no swelling or tenderness. Steady gait without aids. Pedal, radial pulses present. Rapid capillary refill.		✓	✓	✓
Activity (describe)		bed rest	OOB in chair	bed rest
Nurse's signature and title		Jane Doe, RN	Jane Doe, RN	Jane Doe, RN

Only document exceptions to the norm or significant information about the patient.

Key: ✓ Meets assessment criteria

(continued)

Face facts with FACT charting (continued)

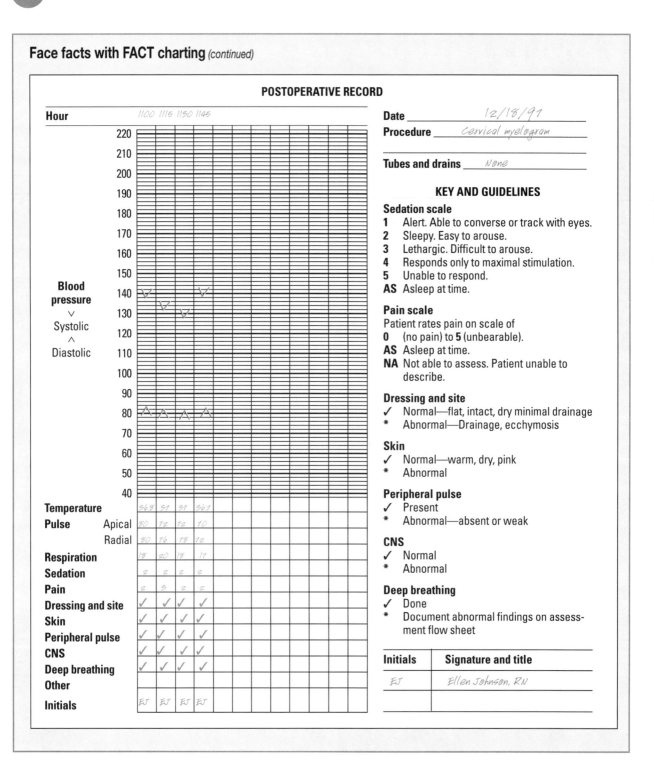

POSTOPERATIVE RECORD

Hour	1100	1115	1130	1145

Blood pressure

∨ Systolic
∧ Diastolic

	1100	1115	1130	1145
Temperature	36.8	37	37	36.7
Pulse — Apical	80	12	12	10
Pulse — Radial	80	16	18	12
Respiration	18	20	18	17
Sedation	2	2	2	2
Pain	2	3	2	2
Dressing and site	✓	✓	✓	✓
Skin	✓	✓	✓	✓
Peripheral pulse	✓	✓	✓	✓
CNS	✓	✓	✓	✓
Deep breathing	✓	✓	✓	✓
Other				
Initials	EJ	EJ	EJ	EJ

Date _____ 12/18/97

Procedure _____ Cervical myelogram

Tubes and drains _____ None

KEY AND GUIDELINES

Sedation scale
1. Alert. Able to converse or track with eyes.
2. Sleepy. Easy to arouse.
3. Lethargic. Difficult to arouse.
4. Responds only to maximal stimulation.
5. Unable to respond.
AS Asleep at time.

Pain scale
Patient rates pain on scale of
0 (no pain) to **5** (unbearable).
AS Asleep at time.
NA Not able to assess. Patient unable to describe.

Dressing and site
✓ Normal—flat, intact, dry minimal drainage
* Abnormal—Drainage, ecchymosis

Skin
✓ Normal—warm, dry, pink
* Abnormal

Peripheral pulse
✓ Present
* Abnormal—absent or weak

CNS
✓ Normal
* Abnormal

Deep breathing
✓ Done
* Document abnormal findings on assessment flow sheet

Initials	Signature and title
EJ	Ellen Johnson, RN

Assessment and action flow sheet

Use the assessment and action flow sheet to document on-going assessments and interventions. Normal assessment parameters for each body system are printed on the form, along with the planned interventions. You may individualize the flow sheet according to the patient's needs.

Frequent assessment flow sheet

The frequent assessment flow sheet is where you chart vital signs and frequent assessments. On a surgical unit, for example, this form would include a postoperative assessment section.

Progress notes

The FACT system requires an integrated progress record. Use narrative notes to document the patient's progress and any significant incidents. As in focus charting, write narrative notes using the data-action-response method. Update progress notes related to patient outcomes every 48 hours.

Advantages of FACT

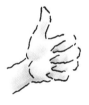

The fact is, the FACT charting system has many good points. For example, this system:
• eliminates repetition and encourages consistent language and structure.
• eliminates detailed charting of normal findings and incorporates each step of the nursing process.
• is outcome oriented and communicates patient progress to all health care team members.
• permits immediate recording of current data and is readily accessible at the patient's bedside.
• eliminates the need for many different forms and reduces the time spent writing narrative notes.

Disadvantages of FACT

FACT charting does have some problems, however, including:
• Development of standards and implementation of a facility-wide system requires a major time commitment.
• Narrative notes may be sketchy, and the nurse's perspective on the patient may be overlooked.
• The nursing process framework may be difficult to identify.

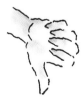

Core charting system

The Core system focuses on the nursing process, which is the core of documentation. It's most useful in acute care and long-term care facilities.

Core framework

This system requires you to assess and record a patient's functional and cognitive status within 8 hours of admission. It consists of the following:
- database
- plan of care
- flow sheets
- progress notes
- discharge summary.

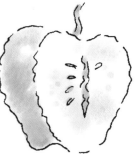

Database

The database (initial assessment form) focuses on the patient's body systems and activities of daily living. It includes a summary of his problems and appropriate nursing diagnoses. The nurse enters the completed database onto the patient's medical record card or Kardex.

Plan of care

The completed plan of care (like the database) goes on the patient's medical record card or Kardex.

Flow sheets

Use flow sheets to document the patient's activities and his response to nursing interventions, diagnostic procedures, and patient teaching.

Progress notes

On the progress notes sheet, record the DAE — that's data (D), action (A), and evaluation (E) or response — for each problem.

Discharge summary

The discharge summary includes information about the nursing diagnoses, patient teaching, and recommended follow-up care.

Advantages of Core

The Core with DAE charting system has several things going for it. For example:
• It incorporates the entire nursing process.
• The DAE component helps to ensure complete documentation based on the nursing process.
• It encourages concise documenting with minimal repetition.
• It allows the daily recording of psychosocial information.

Disadvantages of Core

Oh no! Core with DAE has a worm (four worms, actually). They are:
• Staff members who are used to other documenting systems may need in-depth training.
• Development of forms may be costly and time-consuming.
• The DAE format doesn't always present information chronologically, making it difficult to quickly perceive the patient's progress.
• The progress notes may not always relate to the plan of care, so you need to monitor carefully to make sure the record shows high-quality care.

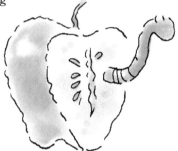

Computerized charting

Computerization can significantly reduce the time you spend on documentation and increase your accuracy. Computers can also be used to help you with other types of paperwork, such as:
• nurse management reports
• patient classification data
• staffing projections.

In addition, they can help you identify patient education needs and supply data for nursing research and education. Some bedside terminals can even measure vital signs.

Besides having a mainframe computer, most health care facilities place personal computers or terminals at workstations throughout the facility so departmental staff will have quick access to vital information. Some facilities put terminals at patients' bedsides, making data even more accessible.

What's the secret code?

Before entering a patient's clinical record onto a computer, you must first enter a special code, which is usually your computer ID number. Some codes may specify the type of information that a particular team member has access to. For example, a dietitian may be assigned a code that allows her to see dietary orders and nutrition histories but not physical therapy information. These codes can help maintain a patient's privacy, unless they're misused.

Cyber-charting

Here's how to use a computerized system for documentation: First, enter the special code, the patient's name, or his account number to bring the patient's electronic chart to the screen. Then choose the function you want to perform.

For example, you can enter new data on the nursing plan of care or progress notes or scan the record to compare data on vital signs or intake and output. Usually, you can obtain information more quickly with computers than with traditional documentation systems.

Computer systems and functions

Depending on which type of computer and software your facility has, you may access information by using your voice, a keyboard, light pen, touch-sensitive screen, or mouse.

Specialized nursing information systems can increase your efficiency in all phases of documentation. Most provide a menu of words or phrases you can choose from to individualize your charting on standardized forms.

With some systems, you can use a series of phrases to quickly create a complete narrative note. Then you can elaborate on a problem or clarify flow sheet documentation in the comment section of a computerized form by entering standardized phrases or typing in comments. Important developments in computer systems include specialized nursing information systems (NIS), the nursing minimum data set (NMDS), and voice activated systems. (See *Computers speed up the nursing process*.)

So, you're my new partner in charting.

I can't waste time

Computers speed up the nursing process

A computer information system can either stand alone or be a subsystem of a larger hospital system. Nursing information systems (NIS) can increase efficiency and accuracy in all phases of the nursing process — assessment, nursing diagnosis, planning, implementation, and evaluation — and can help nurses meet the standards established by the ANA and the JCAHO. In addition, an NIS can help you spend more time meeting the patient's needs. Consider the following uses of computers in the nursing process.

Assessment

Use the computer terminal to record admission information. As you collect data, enter further information as prompted by the computer's software program. Enter data about the patient's health status, history, chief complaint, and other assessment factors.

I'll help you increase efficiency and accuracy!

Some software programs prompt you to ask specific questions and then offer pathways to gather further information. In some systems, if you enter an assessment value that's outside the usual acceptable range, the computer will flag the entry to call your attention to it.

Nursing diagnosis

Most current programs list standard diagnoses with associated signs and symptoms as references. But you must still use clinical judgment to determine a nursing diagnosis for each patient. With this information, you can rapidly obtain diagnostic information.

For example, the computer can generate a list of possible diagnoses for a patient with selected signs and symptoms, or it may enable you to retrieve and review the patient's records according to the nursing diagnosis.

Planning

To help nurses begin writing a plan of care, newer computer programs display recommended expected outcomes and interventions for the selected diagnoses. Computers can also track outcomes for large patient populations.

You can use computers to compare large amounts of patient data, help identify outcomes the patient is likely to achieve based on individual problems and needs, and estimate the time frame for reaching outcome goals.

Implementation

Use the computer to record actual interventions and patient-processing information, such as transfer and discharge instructions, and to communicate this information to other departments. Computer-generated progress notes automatically sort and print out patient data — such as medication administration, treatments, and vital signs — making documentation more efficient and accurate.

Evaluation

During evaluation, use the computer to record and store observations, patient responses to nursing interventions, and your own evaluation statements. You may also use information from other members of the health care team to determine future actions and discharge planning. If a desired patient outcome has not been achieved, record new interventions taken to ensure desired outcomes. Then reevaluate the second set of interventions.

Nursing information systems

Currently available NIS software programs allow you to record nursing actions in the electronic record, making documentation easier. These systems reflect most or all of the components of the nursing process so they can meet the standards of the American Nurses' Association (ANA) and JCAHO.

What's more, each NIS provides different features and can be customized to conform to a facility's documentation forms and formats.

At present, most NISs manage information passively. That is, they collect, transmit, organize, format, print, and display information that you can use to make a decision, but they don't suggest decisions for you. (See *Computerized give and take.*)

Nursing minimum data set

The NMDS program attempts to standardize nursing information. It contains three categories of data:
• nursing care, such as nursing diagnoses and interventions
• patient demographics, such as the patient's name, birth date, gender, race and ethnicity, and residence
• service elements such as length of hospitalization.

What NMDS can do

The NMDS charting system allows you to collect nursing diagnosis and intervention data and identify the nursing needs of various patient populations. It lets you track patient outcomes and describe nursing care in different settings, including the patient's home. It also helps establish accurate estimates for nursing service costs and provides data about nursing care that may influence health care policy and decision making.

Comparing trends

In addition, you can compare nursing trends locally, regionally, and nationally and compare nursing data from various clinical settings, patient populations, and geographic areas.

Better care through better charting

The NMDS also helps you provide better patient care. For instance, examining the outcomes of patient popula-

---

Computerized give and take

The most recent nursing information systems interact with you, prompting you with questions and suggestions about the information you enter. Ultimately, this computerized, sequential decision-making format should lead to more effective nursing care and documentation.

An interactive system requires you to enter only a brief narrative. The questions and suggestions the computer program provides make your documentation thorough and quick. The program also allows you to add or change information so that your documentation fits your patient.

O.K. Let's discuss this.

tions will help you set realistic outcomes for an individual patient. This system also can help you develop accurate nursing diagnoses and plan interventions.

The standardized format encourages more consistent nursing documentation. All data are coded, making documentation and information retrieval faster and easier. Currently, NANDA assigns numerical codes to all nursing diagnoses so they can be used with the NMDS.

Talk to me...

Voice-activated systems

Some facilities have voice-activated nursing documentation systems. These are most useful in departments that have a high volume of structured reports such as the operating room.

This system uses a specialized knowledge base of nursing words, phrases, and report forms, combined with automated speech recognition technology. You can record nurses' notes by voice, promptly and completely. The system requires little or no keyboard use — you simply speak into a telephone handset, and the text appears on the computer screen.

Triggering text

The software program includes information on the nursing process, nursing theory, nursing standards of practice, and report forms in a logical format. Trigger phrases cue the system to display passages of report text. You can use the text displayed to design an individualized plan of care or to fill in standard hospital forms.

Although voice-activated systems work most efficiently with trigger phrases, word-for-word dictation and editing are possible. The system increases the nurse's recording speed and decreases paperwork.

Pros of computer charting

Most nurses have good things to say about computerized charting. For example:
• It makes storing and retrieving information fast and easy.
• You can store data on patient populations that can help improve the quality of nursing care.
• You can efficiently and constantly update information and help link diverse sources of patient information.

• It uses standard terminology, which improves communication among health care disciplines and promotes more accurate comparisons.
• The charting is always legible.
• You can send request slips and patient information from one terminal to another quickly and efficiently, which helps ensure confidentiality.

Cons of computer charting

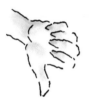

People also have gripes about computer charting, including:
• If used incorrectly, the computer may scramble patient information.
• Computerized charting can threaten patient confidentiality if security measures are neglected.
• The use of standardized phrases and a limited vocabulary can make information inaccurate or incomplete.
• Some people have trouble adjusting to computers, thus increasing the margin for error.
• When the system goes "down," information is temporarily unavailable.
• Computer charting can take extra time if too many nurses try to chart on too few terminals.
• Implementing a computerized documentation system is expensive.

Choosing a charting system

Health care facilities are always striving for greater efficiency and quality of care. A top-notch charting system can help a facility reach these goals.

Remember, documentation is often examined to make sure a facility meets the profession's minimum acceptable level of care. If efficiency and quality levels are low, your charting system may need to be modified or replaced. (See *Does your charting system measure up?*)

Getting better and better

Continuous quality improvement programs are mandated by the state and JCAHO. Committees that set up these programs choose well-defined, objective, and easily measurable indicators that help them assess the structure, process, and outcome of patient care. They also use these

Art of the chart

Does your charting system measure up?

How useful is your current charting system? Is it incomplete, disorganized, or confusing? If so, it won't stand up to later scrutiny in case of a lawsuit or formal review.

To evaluate your charting system, ask yourself the following questions. If you answer no to any of them, you might recommend a closer evaluation of your system.

Documenting interventions and patient progress

• Does your current system reflect the patient's progress and the interventions based on recorded evaluations? Look for records that describe the patient's progress, actual interventions, and evaluations of provided care.

• Does the record include evidence of the patient's response to nursing care? For example, does it report the effectiveness of analgesics or the patient's response to I.V. medications? Does it show that care was modified according to the patient's response to treatment? For example, does it show what action was taken if the patient tolerated only half of a prescribed tube feeding?

• Does the record note continuity of care, or do unexplained gaps appear? If gaps appear, are notes entered later that document previous happenings? If late entries appear in the nurses' notes on subsequent days, do you have to check the entire record to validate care?

• Are daily activities documented? For example, do the notes include evidence that the patient bathed himself or indicate that the patient could independently transfer himself to a wheelchair?

Documenting the health care team's actions

• Does the record portray the nursing process clearly? Look for actual nursing diagnoses, written assessments, interventions, and evaluation of the patient's responses to them.

• Does the current documentation system facilitate and show communication among health care team members? Check for evidence that telephone calls were made, that doctors were paged and notified of changes in a patient's condition, and that actions reflected these communications.

• Is discharge planning clearly documented? Do the records show evidence of interdisciplinary coordination, team conferences, completed patient teaching, and discharge instructions?

• Does the record reflect current standards of care? Does it indicate that caregivers and administrators follow facility policies and procedures? If not, does the system provide for explanations of why a policy wasn't implemented or was implemented in a different way?

Checking for clarity and comprehensiveness

• Are all portions of the record complete? Are all flow sheets, checklists, and other forms completed according to facility policy? Are all necessary entries apparent on the medication forms? If not, does the record describe why a medication wasn't given as ordered and who was informed of the omission if necessary?

• Does the documentation make sense? Can you track the patient's care and hospital course on this record alone?

indicators to monitor and evaluate the contents of a patient's medical record.

Does your charting measure up?

Both shorter hospital stays and the requirement to verify the need for supplies and equipment have placed greater emphasis on nursing documentation as a yardstick for measuring the quality of patient care and determining if it was required and provided.

To verify that treatment was required and provided or that medical tests and supplies were used, the insurers (also called third-party payers) review nursing documentation carefully. As a result, nurses now need to document more information than ever before, including every I.V. needle used to start an infusion, each use of an I.V. pump to deliver a specific volume of medication, and every test that the patient undergoes.

You may be on a committee

When changes are called for, you may be asked to serve on a committee that decides whether your charting system needs a simple revision or total overhaul. Before committing to a totally new system, your committee will discuss the possibility of revising the current system. This, of course, is easier than switching to a new system and changing the way information is collected, entered, and retrieved. (See *To change or not to change*.)

When choosing a new charting system, consider the type of care that's provided at your facility. For example, some systems work better in acute care than in long-term care settings.

Cost is another important factor to consider. Although computer systems are used in almost every care setting, the cost of a new system can be astronomical. All the more reason to weigh the options very carefully.

If a new charting system *is* selected, staff will require plenty of training. The system may be initiated on one unit at a time to make the transition easier.

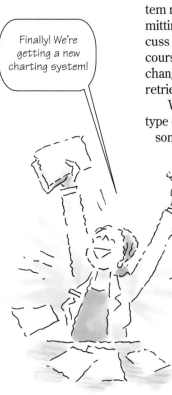

Finally! We're getting a new charting system!

To change or not to change

...that is the question...

Whether you're selecting a new charting system or modifying an existing one, ponder the following questions:
• What are the specific positive features of our current charting system?
• What are the specific problems or limitations of our current system? How can they be resolved?
• How much time will we need to develop a new system, educate the staff, and implement the changes?
• Will a new system be cost effective?
• How will changing the charting system affect other members of the health care team, including the business office staff and medical staff?
• How will we handle resistance to the proposed changes?

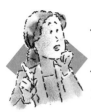

Quick quiz

1. The PIE charting format is useful in:
    A. acute care settings.
    B. long-term care settings.
    C. home care settings.

Answer: A. Patients in long-term care and home care usually aren't acutely ill, so they don't need to be assessed every 8 hours, which PIE requires. Doing so would generate lengthy, repetitious notes.

2. A disadvantage of POMR documentation is its emphasis on:
    A. the priority of problems.
    B. the chronology of problems.
    C. SOAP notes.

Answer: B. When the emphasis is put on chronology instead of priority, teammates may disagree about which problems to list.

3. An advantage of narrative documentation is:
    A. it clearly tracks trends and problems.
    B. it's flexible in various clinical settings.
    C. it uses flow charts.

Answer: B. The most flexible of all charting systems, narrative charting suits any clinical setting and strongly conveys your nursing interventions and your patients' responses.

4. In the Core (with DAE) charting system, DAE stands for:
    A. date, activity, emotional status.
    B. data, assessment, expected outcomes.
    C. data, action, evaluation.

Answer: C. This information is recorded on the progress sheet for each problem.

5. When deciding which charting system to use, give the least consideration to:
    A. your geographical area.
    B. legal issues.
    C. professional standards.

Answer: A. Health care facilities also consider accrediting requirements when deciding which charting system would be the most effective.

6. An important factor to consider when evaluating your current documentation system is:
   A.   Will the staff complain if you decide to change it?
   B.   Does the record include evidence of the patient's response to nursing care?
   C.   Has it become second nature because you've used it so long?

Answer: B. An incomplete, disorganized, or confusing record won't stand up to legal scrutiny or formal review. Learning a new system is time consuming, but it's well worth the effort.

Scoring

☆☆☆   If you answered all six items correctly, be careful. You're doing so much charting, you risk getting "narrative note elbow!"

☆☆   If you answered four or five correctly, three cheers! You have an uncanny aptitude for filling in the blanks in a standardized care plan!

☆   If you answered fewer than four correctly, don't fret! You will have plenty of opportunities to document your way to distinction, using narrative notes, the problem-oriented medical record, the PIE system, Focus charting, CBE, the FACT system, computerized charting....

Part II

Charting in contemporary health care

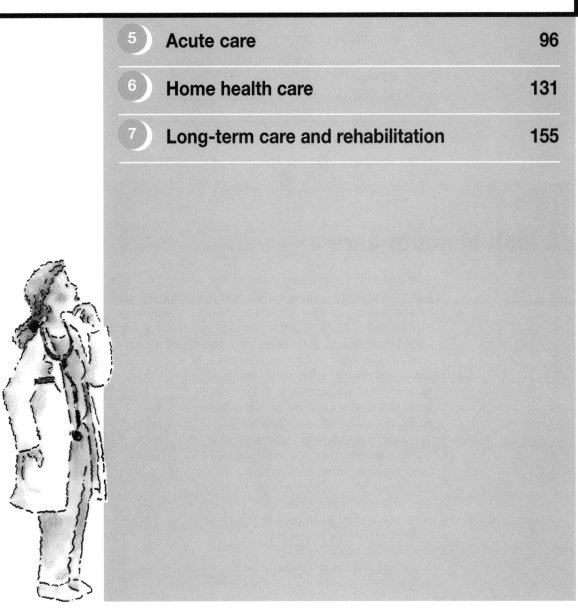

Acute care

Just the facts

In this chapter you'll learn:

♦ what medical record forms are used in acute care settings

♦ the contents and organization of those forms

♦ the advantages and disadvantages of each medical record form

♦ more detailed information about critical pathways.

A look at acute care

Like many nurses working in acute care settings, you may feel discouraged — even overwhelmed — by the amount of information you have to document each day. You may also be baffled by new methods of documentation, such as computer charting, flow sheets, and critical pathways. Ironically, formats that are meant to save time for nurses may actually end up costing more time. Nurses accustomed to writing long, handwritten notes may be uncomfortable taking advantage of "shortcuts" offered by newer methods, especially in today's litigious environment where documentation is strongly linked to liability. The result: Many nurses end up double documenting, for example, recording the information with a check mark on a flow sheet and then documenting it again longhand in progress notes.

> Nurses uncomfortable with newer methods of charting may wind up double documenting.

To cope with the documentation chaos that characterizes contemporary nursing, your best weapon is familiarity with the variety of formats available, their advantages and disadvantages, and how you can use them to enhance your nursing practice.

Forms, forms, and more forms

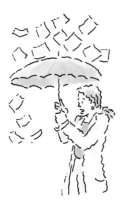

The following forms — commonly used to create medical records in acute care settings — are explained in this chapter:
- admission database or admission assessment forms
- nursing plans of care
- critical pathways
- patient care Kardexes
- graphic forms
- progress notes
- flow sheets
- discharge summary and patient discharge instruction forms.

Other forms include patient-teaching documents, dictated documentation, and patient self-documentation. Adapted or newly developed forms also may be used.

Yes, these forms do serve a purpose

A medical record with well-organized, completed forms serves three purposes:

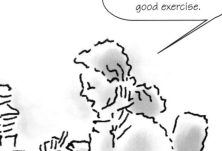

A purpose for these forms? Well, for one, my wrist gets good exercise.

It helps you to communicate patient information to other members of the health care team.

It protects you and your employer legally, by providing evidence of the nature and quality of care the patient received.

It's used by your facility to obtain accreditation and reimbursement for care.

In the long run, taking the time to carefully commit patient information to a standard, easy-to-use format frees you to spend more time on direct patient care.

Admission database form

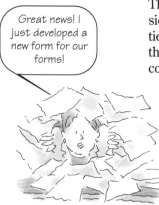

Great news! I just developed a new form for our forms!

The admission database form — also known as an admission assessment — is used to document your initial patient assessment. The scope of information documented at this stage is usually broad because you're establishing a comprehensive base of clinical information.

The admission assessment — including a health history and physical examination — must be completed within 24 hours of admission, unless a shorter time frame is required by your facility. To complete the admission database form, you must collect relevant information from various sources and analyze it. The finished form portrays a complete picture of the patient at admission.

The form of the form

The admission database form may be organized in different ways. Some facilities use a form organized by body system. Others use a format that groups information to reflect principles of nursing practice such as patient response patterns.

Nursing-medical mixer

More and more facilities are using integrated admission database forms. On integrated admission database forms, nursing and medical assessments complement each other, reducing the need for repeated documentation. (See *Integrated admission database form.*)

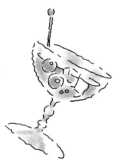

Charting with style

Regardless of how the form is organized, findings are documented in two basic styles:

☞ standardized, open-ended style, which comes with preprinted headings and questions

✌ standardized, closed-ended style, which has preprinted headings, checklists, and questions with specific responses (you simply check off the appropriate response). Most facilities use a combination of different styles in one form.

(Text continues on page 103.)

Art of the chart

Integrated admission database form

Most health care facilities use a multidisciplinary admission form. The sample form below has spaces that can be filled in by the nurse, doctor, and other health care providers.

Name _Beatrice Perry_

Address _2 Clayton Street_
Dallas, Texas

Admission Date _12_/_27_/_91_ Time _1345_

Admitted per: ___ Ambulatory
✔ Stretcher ___ Wheelchair

T _97_ P _92_ R _24_ BP _98_ / _52_

Ht. _5'2"_ Wt. _225 lb_
(estimated/actual)

ORIENTATION TO ROOM/UNIT POLICIES EXPLAINED
✔ Call light
✔ Bed oper.
✔ Phone
✔ Television
✔ Meals
___ Advance directive explained

___ Valuables form c[...]
___ Elec.
___ Smoking
✔ Side rails
___ ID bracelet on
✔ Visiting hours

> Be time-efficient by asking technicians or nursing assistants to get some information.

SECTION COMPLETED BY: _K. Crawford CST_ **TIME:** _1350_

Name and phone numbers of two people to call if necessary:

NAME	RELATIONSHIP	PHONE#
Mary Ryan	daughter	665-2190
John Carr	son	665-4185

REASON FOR HOSPITALIZATION ___ (patient quote:) _I go numb in my rt. arm and leg_

ANTICIPATED DATE OF DISCHARGE: _12/30/91_

PREVIOUS HOSPITALIZATIONS: SURGERY/ILLNESS   DATE
TIA   _11/4/91_

HEALTH PROBLEM	Yes	No	?
Arthritis		✔	
Blood problem (anemia, sickle cell, clotting, bleeding)		✔	
Cancer		✔	
Diabetes	✔		
Eye problems (cataracts, glaucoma)		✔	
Heart problem		✔	
Liver problem		✔	
Hiatal hernia		✔	
High blood pressure	✔		
HIV/AIDS		✔	
Kidney problem		✔	
Comments:			

HEALTH PROBLEM	Yes	No	?
Lung problem (Emphysema, Asthma, Bronchitis, TB, Pneumonia, Shortness of breath)	✔		
Stroke		✔	
Ulcers		✔	
Thyroid problem		✔	
Psychological disorder		✔	
Alcohol abuse		✔	
Drug abuse			
Drug(s)_____		✔	
Smoking	✔		
Other _____			

ALLERGIES: ☐ TAPE ☐ IODINE ☐ LATEX ☐ no known allergies
☐ FOOD:_____ ☑ DRUG: _Penicillin_
☐ BLOOD REACTION:_____ ☐ OTHER:_____

MEDICATIONS: _____

INFORMATION RECEIVED FROM: **SECTION COMPLETED BY:**
☑ Patient ☐ Relative_____ ☐ Friend_____ ☐ Other_____ _N. O'Meara, RN_ Date _12/27/91_ Time _1405_

(continued)

Integrated admission database form (continued)

This diagram allows you to map any impairment in skin integrity.

All assessment sections are to be completed by a professional nurse. Date 12/21/91

GENERAL PHYSICAL APPEARANCE

✓ Clean _____ Disheveled

SKIN INTEGRITY: Indicate the location of any of the following on the chart to the right using the designated letter: a = rashes, b = lesions, c = significant bruises/abrasions, d = burns, e = pressure sores, f = recent scars, g = presence of tubes/appliances, h = other

Comments: b= ischemic leg ulcers (2cm - healing)

PRESSURE SORE POTENTIAL ASSESSMENT

PARAMETERS	0	1	2	3	Score
Mental status	(Alert)	Lethargic	Semi-Comatose	Comatose	0
			Count These Conditions As Double		
Activity	Ambulatory	(Needs help)	Chairfast	Bedfast	1
Mobility	Full	(Limited)	Very limited	Immobile	1
Incontinence	(None)	Occasional	Usually of urine	Total of urine and feces	0
Oral nutrition intake	Good	(Fair)	Poor	None	1
Oral fluid intake	(Good)	Fair	Poor	None	0
Predisposing diseases (diabetes, neuropathies, vascular disease, anemias)	Absent	Slight	Moderate	(Severe)	6
Patients with scores of 10 or above should be considered at risk.				Total	9

FALL-RISK ASSESSMENT

Impaired: ____sensory function
____urinary/GI function
____mobility function
____mental status
____general debility/weakness
✓history of recent falls/dizziness/blackouts (automatically designates patient as prone-to-fall)
✓Prone-to-fall risk (indicated on nursing Kardex _____✓___)

NEUROLOGICAL

____Dizziness ____Syncope ____Headache ____Blurred vision
____Recent seizure ✓Numbness/tingling location: Rt. arm and leg
LOC: ✓Alert ____Lethargic ____Semi-comatose ____Comatose
Mental Status: ✓Oriented ____Confused ____Disoriented
Speech: ✓Clear ____Slurred ____Garbled ____Aphasic

Neurological Checklist

Right Arm	Right Leg	R.Pupil	Coma Scale					
Left Arm	Left Leg	L. Pupil	Pupil Reaction	Eyes Open	Best Verbal Response	Best Motor Response	Total	
12/14	12/14	5/6	1	4	5	6	15	

	Response	1	2	3	4	5	6
COMA SCALE CODE	EYES OPEN	Never	To Pain	To Sound	Sponta-neously		
	VERBAL	None	Incompre-hensible Sounds	Inappro-priate words	Confused Conversa-tion	Oriented	
	MOTOR	None	Extension	Flexion Abnormal	Flexion Withdrawal	Localizes Pain	

+1:cannot move
+2:cannot move against gravity
+3:move against gravity
+4:move strongly against gravity

Comments: numbness transient

T. Jones, MD

CODE
Pupils:
mm

Extremities movement/strength
Pupil Reaction
- Reactive
- Nonreactive
D Dilated
C Constricted
> Greater than
< Less than
= Equal
= Sluggish

1 •
2 •
3 •
4 ●
5 ●
6 ●
7 ⬤

BEHAVIORAL

Behavior: ✓Cooperative ____Uncooperative ____Depressed ____Restless
____Combative ✓Anxious ____Unresponsive ____Other _____
Comments: _____
Religious/Spiritual beliefs: Lutheran
P. request to contact minister/priest/rabbi? ✓Y ____N
Name Reverend Thomas Jones Phone # 555-4192

These circles will help you document pupil reaction accurately.

Integrated admission database form *(continued)*

Addressograph	Date *12/27/91*

CARDIOVASCULAR

Skin Color: ___Normal ___Flushed ___Pale ✔Cyanotic
Apical Pulse: ___Regular ✔Irregular ___Pacemaker: Type _____ Rate _____
Peripheral Pulses: ✔Present ___Equal ✔Weak ___Absent Comments: *bilat. weak lower extremities*
Specify: R___radial ___pedal L ___radial ___pedal
Comments:_____
Edema: ___No ✔Yes *+1 bilat. pretibial* Numbness: ___No ✔Yes Site:_*Rt. arm and leg*_
Chest Pain: ✔No ___Yes___ P_____ Q_____ R_____ S_____ T_____
Family Cardiac History: ___No ✔Yes Telemetry Monitor: ___No ✔Yes rhythm_*normal sinus*_
Comments:_____

PULMONARY

Respirations: ✔Regular ___Irregular ___Shortness of breath ___Dyspnea on exertion
O₂ use at home? ___Yes ✔No
Chest expansion: ✔Symmetrical ___Asymmetrical (explain: _____)
Breath sounds: ___Clear ___Crackles ___Rhonchi ✔Wheezing Location *bilat upper lobe, inspiratory*
Cough: None ✔Nonproductive ___Productive ___ Describe _____
Comments:_*pulse oximetry 98% on 2 L; sleeps with 2 pillows*_

GASTROINTESTINAL

Stool: ✔Formed Diarrhea ___ Obese ✔ *NUTRITION:
___Loose Constipation ___ thin ___ ✔Special Diet
___Liquid Abdomen: ✔Soft emaciated ___ *1800 ADA*
___Mucus ___Rigid nourished ___ ___Tube feeding
___Ostomy ✔Nontender ___Chewing problem
___Incontinent ___Tender ___Swallowing problems
Color: ✔Brown ___(Location) ___Nausea/vomiting
___Black Bowel Sounds ✔Present ___Poor appetite
___Red tinged ___Absent ___Wt. loss/gain ___ lb
___Bloody ___Hypoactive
___Hyperactive *** Refer to dietitian if any ✔**

GENITOURINARY/REPRODUCTIVE

Color of Urine: ✔Yellow ___Amber ___Pink/Red tinged ___Brown ___Orange ___Clear ___Cloudy
___Ileo-Conduit ___Incontinent ___Catheter in place ___Frequency ___Urgency
___Difficulty in initiating stream ___Pain ___Burning ___Oliguria ___Anuria
___Dialysis Access site: _____ Date of last Dialysis: _____
Comments:_____
Date of LMP _*1977*_ Date of last PAP _*5/95*_ Breast self-exam ___Yes ✔No
Use of contraceptives: ___Yes (type _____) ___No ✔N/A
   Vaginal Discharge: ___Yes (describe _____) ✔No
   Bleeding: ___Yes (amount _____) ✔No
Pregnancies: Pregnant ___Yes ___Weeks gravida ___ Para ___ ✔No
Date of last Prostate Exam _____ Testicular self-exam ___Yes ___No
Comments: _____

ACTIVITY/MOBILITY PATTERNS

___Ambulates independently ___Full ROM ___Limited ROM (explain: _____)
✔Ambulates with assistance (explain:_____) ✔cane ___walker ___crutches
___Gait steady/unsteady ___Mobility in bed (ability to turn self) _____
Musculoskeletal ___ Pain___ Weakness___ Contractures___ Joint swelling
___ Paralysis___ Deformity___ Joint stiffness___ Cast___ Amputation
Describe: _____
Comments: _____

REST/SLEEP PATTERNS

___ Use of sleeping aids _____ Sleeps _*6*_ hr/day
Comments:_____

Additional assessment comment: _*On arrival, diaphoretic and ⊕ hand tremors. vital signs stable. glucose 56 mg/dl.*_
Orange juice and lunch given to pt. 2 hr postprandial glucose 204. Symptoms subsided with juice. Nutrition and diabetes
educator consulted. ——————————————————— *N. O'Meara, RN*
MRI shows no cerebral lesions. carotid doppler ultrasound pending. ——————— *T. Jones, MD*

> Note that room is provided for additional comments.

(continued)

Integrated admission database form *(continued)*

> This final page deals with patient teaching and discharge planning.

EDUCATION/DISCHARGE SECTION
Instructions: Assessment sections must be completed within 8 hours of admission. Discharge planning and summary must be completed by day of discharge.

Addressograph

EDUCATIONAL ASSESSMENT

Yes	No	
✓		Patient understands current diagnosis
✓		Family/significant other understands diagnosis
✓		Patient able to read English
✓		Patient able to write English
✓		Patient able to communicate
	✓	Patient/family understands pre-hospital medication/treatment regimen

Yes	No	Emotional Factors:
✓		Patient appears to be coping*
✓		Family appears to be coping*
	✓	Any suspicion of family violence
	✓	Any suspicion of family abuse
	✓	Any suspicion of family neglect

Comment: _diabetic teaching_

Language spoken, written, and read (other than English): _____
Interpreter services needed: ✓No ___Yes
Are there any barriers to learning (e.g., emotional, physical, cognitive)? _No_
Religious or cultural practices that may alter care or teaching needs? ___Yes ✓No Describe: _____
Is pt/family motivated to learn? ✓Yes ___No describe: _____

> This assessment form is multidisciplinary. In this example, both nurses and doctors provided information.

DISCHARGE ASSESSMENT

Living arrangements/caregiver (relationship): _lives alone_
Type of dwelling: ___Apartment ✓House ___Nursing Home ___More than 1 floor? ✓Yes___No Describe: _____
___Boarding Home ___Other _____
Physical barriers in home: ✓No ___Yes (explain: _____
Access to follow-up medical care: ✓Yes ___No (explain: _____
Ability to carry out ADL: ___Self-care ✓Partial assistance ___Total assistance
Needs help with: ✓Bathing ___Feeding ___Ambulation ___Other _____
Anticipated discharge destination: ___Home ___Rehab. ✓Nursing Home ___SNF ___Boarding Home _____
___Other _____
Currently receiving services from a community agency? ___ Yes ___No
  If yes, check which one ___visiting nurses ___Meals on Wheels
Concerned about returning home? ___Being alone ___Financial problems ___Homemaking ___Meal prep.
___Managing ADLs ___Other _____

Assessment completed by: _N. O'Meara, RN_ Date _12/21/91_ Time _1430_
Assessment completed by: _T. Jones, MD_ Date _12/21/91_ Time _1445_

DISCHARGE PLANNING

Resources notified:	Name	Date	Time	Signature
Social worker				
Home care coordinator	M. Murphy, RN	12/28/91	0900	
Other_____				

Equipment/Supplies needed: _stair chair_
Arranged for by: _M. Murphy, RN_ Date _12/28/91_ Time _0930_
Comment: _daughter to stay with pt at home_

DISCHARGE SUMMARY

Alterations in patterns: If yes, explain.	Yes	No	Explanation
Nutrition	✓		adherence to ADA diet regimen
Elimination		✓	
Self-care		✓	
Skin integrity		✓	
Mobility	✓		needs help with stairs
Comfort pain		✓	
Mental status/behavior		✓	
Vision/Hearing/Speech		✓	

Discharge instructions given (specify): _standard hosp. discharge instruction sheet_
Effects of illness on employment/lifestyle: _____
Central venous line removed: _N/A_ By Whom: _____
Belongings sent with patient: ✓clothes ✓dentures ✓eyeglasses ___ hearing aid ___ prosthesis ___ valuables
✓prescriptions ✓other _cane_
Follow-up medical supervision to be provided by: _Dr. Gehran_
✓Patient/family instructed to call for follow-up appointment Discharge destination: _pt's home with daughter_
Section completed by: _C. Rafferty, RN_ Date _12/30/91_ Time _1215_

As you complete the admission database form, keep in mind that the information you chart is used by the Joint Commission on Accreditation of Healthcare Organizations (JCAHO), quality improvement groups, and other parties to continue accreditation, justify requests for reimbursement, and maintain or improve patient care standards.

> The wealth of information gathered during admission is amazing!

The function of the form

A carefully completed admission database form is extremely valuable. It contains physiologic, psychosocial, and cultural information that's useful throughout the patient's stay in your facility. It contains:
- baseline data that's used later for comparison with the patient's progress
- important information about the patient's current health status as well as clues about actual and potential health problems (For example, your admission assessment may turn up facts about prescription and over-the-counter drugs the patient takes; possible drug allergies also may be revealed.)
- insight into the patient's ability to comply with therapy and his expectations for treatments
- details about the patient's lifestyle, family relationships, and cultural influences. (During discharge planning, you'll need information about the patient's living arrangements, caregivers, resources, and support systems.)

How to use the admission database form

Conduct the patient interview and record the information on the admission form or progress notes as soon as possible, noting the date and time of the entry.

Acute illness, short hospital stays, and staff shortages can make it difficult to conduct a thorough and accurate initial interview. In some cases, you can ask the patient to complete a questionnaire about his past and present health status and use this to document his health history.

Ready, willing, and able?

Before completing the admission database form, consider the patient's ability and readiness to participate. For example, if he's sedated, confused, hostile, angry, or having pain or breathing problems, ask only the most essential questions. You can perform an in-depth interview later, when his condition improves.

That's what families are for

If the patient can't provide information, consider seeking help from friends or family members. Be sure to document your source.

During your interview, try to alleviate as much of the patient's discomfort and anxiety as possible. Also, try to create a quiet, private environment for your talk.

If the patient is too ill to be interviewed and family members aren't available, base your initial assessment on your observations and physical examination. *Be sure to document on the admission form why you couldn't obtain complete data.*

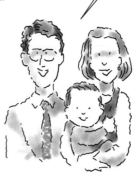

Ask us. We're happy to help.

Potential problems

Admission database forms can present some difficulties. For example:

• Through no fault of your own, you won't be able to complete some forms. The quality of recorded data depends in part on the ability of the patient or members of his family to provide accurate information.

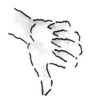

• You may inadvertently chart inaccurate information, especially if the patient is too sick to answer questions or a family member can't answer appropriately for him.

• Many other people will chart on the integrated admission database forms. When using such a form, the risk that information may be missing or incorrect increases. You can't assume that colleagues collected the right information. You are responsible for verifying and correcting information gathered by nursing assistants and LPNs; likewise, the doctor is responsible for verifying information that you have collected. Remember, adding new information later may require you to revise the plan of care accordingly.

Plans of care and critical pathways

In acute care settings today, two different formats are being used to guide the process of care for a patient — the traditional plan of care and the critical pathway. Both formats offer important advantages and disadvantages. The traditional plan of care, based on a nursing assessment and nursing diagnosis, provides a more precise account of the patient's individual nursing needs. The standardized critical pathway is a better tool for facilitating interdisciplinary communication and perhaps more suited to the demands of the managed care environment.

Plans of care

The full nursing care needs of any patient are unlikely to be documented on a critical pathway. For this reason, some acute care facilities are continuing to rely on the traditional format of a plan of care as the chief mechanism for documenting each patient's nursing care.

Documentation guidelines (what else?)

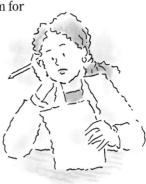

Although JCAHO no longer requires a specific care-planning format, the commission does require that the following information be included in plans of care in an acute care setting:

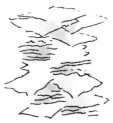
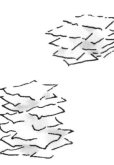

• ongoing assessments of the patient's illness and response to care, including patient needs, concerns, problems, capabilities, and limitations
• ongoing evaluation and modification of nursing diagnoses, interventions, and expected outcomes, based on identified patient needs and care priorities
• notation of nursing interventions, patient monitoring and surveillance, and patient responses
• reevaluation of patient progress compared with goals and the care plan
• documentation of the inability to meet patient care goals and the reason for this
(For more information about plans of care, see Chapter 3, Plans of care.)

Critical pathways

Many acute care facilities are abandoning the traditional plan of care in favor of a standardized critical pathway. Critical pathways are combinations of medical and nursing plans of care.

A time of transition

The changeover from plan to pathway has thrown nursing documentation into a transitional state. You may find yourself working in a facility that uses both formats. Many nurses are not yet comfortable with critical pathways and are double-documenting — copying information from a pathway into a care plan.

Following the pathway

Critical pathways are used in health care facilities that employ case management systems for delivering care. In such a system, a registered nurse acting as case manager oversees a closely monitored and controlled system of multidisciplinary care.

Nurses, doctors, and other health care providers are responsible for establishing a care track, or case map, for each diagnosis-related group (DRG). A DRG is a way of classifying a patient according to his medical diagnosis for the purpose of obtaining reimbursement for hospital costs. The care track is used to determine a patient's daily care requirements and desired outcomes. The average length of stay for the patient's DRG is used in defining the care track. The case manager oversees achievement of outcomes, length of stay, and the use of equipment throughout the patient's illness.

Why take the pathway?

For acute care facilities, critical pathways work best with diagnoses that have fairly predictable outcomes, for example, hip replacement, cerebrovascular accident, myocardial infarction, or open heart surgery. The pathway is a way to standardize and organize care for routine conditions. It makes it easier for the case manager to track data needed to streamline use of materials and human resources, ensure that patients receive quality care, improve coordination of care, and reduce the cost of care.

Health care facilities have a financial incentive to switch to critical pathway documentation. Well-developed critical pathways with demonstrated cost reductions may provide the facility with an advantage when negotiating contracts with managed care organizations.

Precautions along the pathway

Using a critical pathway doesn't eliminate the need for nurses to diagnose and treat human responses to health problems. Patients are individuals and commonly require nursing intervention beyond that specified in the critical pathway.

For example, a patient enters the hospital for a hip replacement and can't communicate verbally because of a previous stroke. The critical pathway wouldn't include measures to assist this patient in making his needs known. Therefore, you would develop a nursing care plan around the nursing diagnosis *Verbal communication impairment.* By using the critical pathway and developing a nursing care plan based on the patient's individual nursing diagnoses, you can provide the best in collaborative care. (For more information about critical pathways, see Chapter 3, Plans of care.)

Patient care Kardex

The patient care Kardex, sometimes called the nursing Kardex, gives a quick overview of basic patient care information. A Kardex typically contains boxes that allow you to check off items that apply to each patient. It also contains space for recording current orders for medications, patient care activities, treatments, and tests. (See *Considering the Kardex,* pages 108 and 109.)

A Kardex isn't a JCAHO requirement. Some facilities have eliminated Kardexes and incorporated the information they contain into the patient's plan of care.

It's all in the Kardex

Refer to the Kardex during change-of-shift reports and throughout the day. It includes the following information:
• the patient's name, age, marital status, and religion — which is usually on the address stamp
• medical diagnoses, listed by priority
• nursing diagnoses, listed by priority
• current doctors' orders for medication, treatments, diet, I.V. therapy, diagnostic tests, procedures, and other measures
• consultations

(Text continues on page 110.)

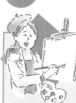

Art of the chart

Considering the Kardex

Here's an example of a patient care Kardex for a medical-surgical unit. Remember that the categories, words, and phrases on a Kardex are brief and intended to trigger images of special circumstances, procedures, activities, or patient conditions.

Care status
Self-care ☐
Partial care with assistance ☐
Complete care ☑
Shower with assistance ☑
Tub ☐
Active exercises ☐
Passive exercises ☐

Special Care
Back care ☑
Mouth care ☑
Foot care ☐
Perineal care ☑
Catheter care ☐
Tracheostomy care ☐
Other (specify)_____ ☐

Condition
Satisfactory ☐
Fair ☐
Guarded ☑
Critical ☐
No code ☐
Advance directive?
    Yes ☑
    No ☐
Date _11/12/91_____

Prosthesis
Dentures
    upper ☑
    lower ☑
Contact lenses ☐
Glasses ☑
Hearing Aid ☑
Other (specify)_____ ☐

Isolation
Strict ☐
Wound and skin ☐
Respiratory ☑
Hepatitis ☐
Enteric ☐
Other (specify)_____ ☐

Diet
Type: _low fat, no conc. sweets_
Force fluids ☐
NPO ☐
Assist with feeding ☐
Isolation tray ☑
Calorie count ☐
Supplements_____

Tube feedings ☐
Type: _____
Rate: _____
Route: _____
    NG ☐
    G tube ☐
    J tube ☐

Admission
Height: _60"_
Weight: _145 lb (61 kg)_
BP: _124/72_
TPR: _100.4 T.P.O. - 92-24_

Frequency
BP: _q shift_
TPR: _q shift_
Apical pulses:
Peripheral pulses: _q shift_
Weight:
Neuro check:
Monitor:
Strips:
Turn:
Cough: _q shift_
Deep breathe: _q shift_
Central venous
    pressure:
Other (specify)_____

GI tubes
Salem syrup ☐
Levin tube ☐
Feeding tube ☐
Type (specify):_____
Other (specify):_____ ☐

Activity
Bed rest ☐
Chair t.i.d. ☑
Dangle ☐
Commode ☐
Commode with assist ☑
Ambulate ☑
BRP ☑
Fall-risk category (specify): _____ ☐
Other (specify):_____ ☐

Mode of transport
Wheelchair ☑
Stretcher ☐
With oxygen ☐

I.V. devices
Heparin lock ☐
Peripheral I.V. ☐
Central line ☑
Triple-lumen CVP ☐
Hickman ☐
Jugular ☐
Peripherally inserted ☐
Parenteral nutrition ☐
Irrigations:_____

Dressings
Type: _CVP_
Change: _q36h_

> The check marks are intended to alert you to important patient care considerations.

Considering the Kardex *(continued)*

> You can quickly find the information you need with this format.

...therapy

SVO$_2$ level (%)
Oxygen ☑
Liters/minute *2 L/minute* ☑
Method
    Nasal cannula ☑
    Face mask ☐
    Venturi (Venti) mask ☐
    Nonrebreather mask ☐
    Trach collar ☐
Nebulizer ☑
Chest PT ☐
Incentive spirometry ☑

> The format and specific information on a Kardex may vary. For instance, the cover sheet of a patient care Kardex on a critical care unit would include the same basic information already shown plus information specific to the unit.

Drains
Type: _____
Number: _____
Location: _____

Urine Output
I&O ☑
Strain urine ☐
Indwelling catheter ☐
Date inserted _____
Size: _____
Intermittent catheter ☐
    Frequency: _____

Side rails
Constant ☐
PRN ☐
Nights ☐

Restraints
Date: _____
Type: _____

Specimens and tests
CBC daily
24-hour collection
Other (specify)_____

Stools
_____

Special notes
_____

Social services
consulted 11/12/91

Monitoring
Hardwire ☐
Telemetry ☑

Pulmonary artery catheter ☐
    Pulmonary artery
    pressure _____
    Pulmonary artery
    wedge pressure: _____
Arterial line ☐
Other (specify) _____ ☐

Mechanical ventilation
Type: _____
Tidal volume: _____
FIO$_2$ _____
Mode: _____
Rate: _____

> On an obstetrics unit, you might find additional information on the Kardex cover sheet.

Delivery
Date: *11/4/91*
Time: *0125*
Type of delivery: *c-section*

Special procedures
Perineal rinse ☐
Sitz bath ☐
Witch hazel compress ☐
Breast binders ☐
Ice ☐
Abdominal binders ☑
Other (specify)_____ ☐

Mother
Due date: _____
Gravida:_____
Para: _____
Rh: _____
Blood type: _____
Membranes ruptured: _____
Episiotomy ☐
Lacerations ☐
RhoGAM studies?
    Yes ☐
    No ☐
Rubella titer?
    Yes ☐
    No ☐

Infant
Male ☐
Female ☐
Full term ☐
Premature ☐
    Weeks ☐
Apgar score ☐
Nursing ☐
Formula ☐
Condition (specify): _____
Other (specify): _____

• results of diagnostic tests and procedures
• permitted activities, functional limitations, assistance
that's needed, and safety precautions.

All shapes and sizes

Kardexes come in various shapes, sizes, and types and
may be computer-generated. Some facilities use different
Kardexes to document specific information, such as medication information, test results, and nonnursing data.

Computerized Kardex

Typically used to record laboratory or diagnostic test results and X-ray findings, a computerized Kardex usually
includes information on medical orders, referrals, consultations, specimens (for culture and sensitivity tests or for
blood glucose analysis, for example), vital signs, diet, and
activity restrictions. (See *Computer-generated patient care
Kardex*.)

Advantages of Kardexes

The Kardex has some good points, including:
• It allows quick access to information about task-orient-
ed interventions, such as specific patient care, medication
administration, and I.V. therapy.
• The plan of care may be added to the Kardex to provide
all the necessary data for patient care, although this dupli-
cates information.

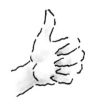

Disadvantages of Kardexes

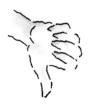

The Kardex has one major drawback: It's only as useful as
nurses make it. It's not an effective charting tool if there
isn't enough space for appropriate information, if it's not
updated frequently, if it's not completed, or if you don't
read it before giving patient care.

In addition, Kardexes are not usually part of the permanent record, so be sure the information on the Kardex
is also found elsewhere on the patient's chart.

How to use the Kardex

The Kardex is most effective when you tailor the information to the needs of a particular setting. For instance, an
intensive care unit Kardex should include information on
hard wire or telemetry monitoring and arterial pressure
monitoring.

Art of the chart

Computer-generated patient care Kardex

In the computer-generated Kardex shown below, you'll find a detailed list of medical orders and other patient care data.

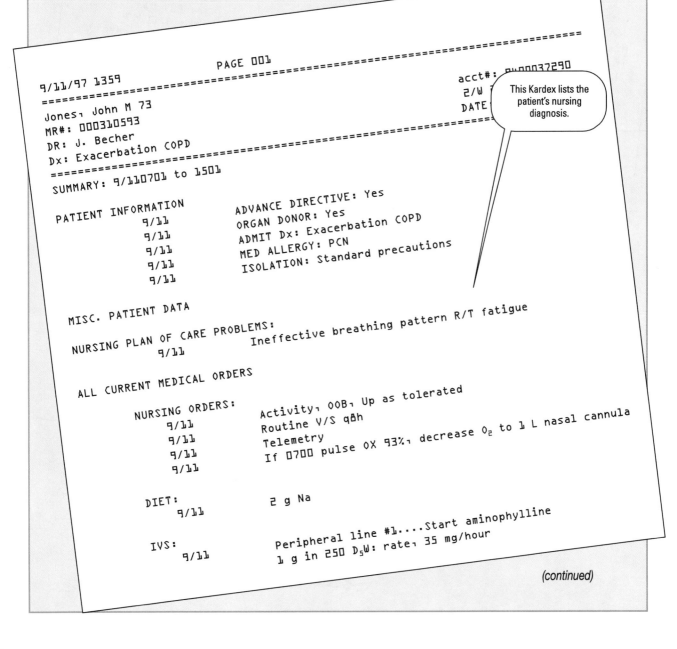

```
                            PAGE 001
9/11/97 1359                                                   acct#: 0000037290
===============================================================   2/W
Jones, John M 73                                              DATE
MR#: 000310593
DR: J. Becher
Dx: Exacerbation COPD
===============================================================
   SUMMARY: 9/110701 to 1501

      PATIENT INFORMATION      ADVANCE DIRECTIVE: Yes
                  9/11        ORGAN DONOR: Yes
                  9/11        ADMIT Dx: Exacerbation COPD
                  9/11        MED ALLERGY: PCN
                  9/11        ISOLATION: Standard precautions
                  9/11


   MISC. PATIENT DATA

   NURSING PLAN OF CARE PROBLEMS:
                  9/11              Ineffective breathing pattern R/T fatigue


   ALL CURRENT MEDICAL ORDERS

         NURSING ORDERS:       Activity, OOB, Up as tolerated
                  9/11        Routine V/S q8h
                  9/11        Telemetry
                  9/11        If 0700 pulse OX 93%, decrease O2 to 1 L nasal cannula
                  9/11

         DIET:                 2 g Na
                  9/11

         IVS:                  Peripheral line #1....Start aminophylline
                  9/11        1 g in 250 D5W: rate, 35 mg/hour
```

This Kardex lists the patient's nursing diagnosis.

(continued)

Computer-generated patient care Kardex *(continued)*

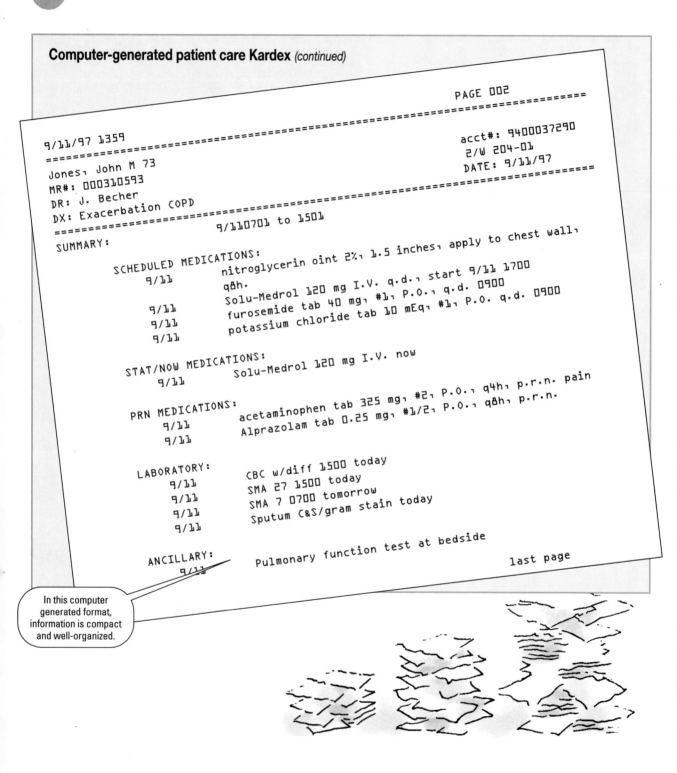

```
                                                        PAGE 002
                                          ==========================
 9/11/97 1359
 ==============================================
                                          acct#: 9400037290
 Jones, John M 73                         2/W 204-01
 MR#: 000310593                           DATE: 9/11/97
 DR: J. Becher                            ==========================
 DX: Exacerbation COPD
 ==============================================
                      9/110701 to 1501
 SUMMARY:

         SCHEDULED MEDICATIONS:
            9/11        nitroglycerin oint 2%, 1.5 inches, apply to chest wall,
                        q8h.
                        Solu-Medrol 120 mg I.V. q.d., start 9/11 1700
            9/11        furosemide tab 40 mg, #1, P.O., q.d. 0900
            9/11        potassium chloride tab 10 mEq, #1, P.O. q.d. 0900
            9/11

         STAT/NOW MEDICATIONS:
            9/11        Solu-Medrol 120 mg I.V. now

         PRN MEDICATIONS:
            9/11        acetaminophen tab 325 mg, #2, P.O., q4h, p.r.n. pain
            9/11        Alprazolam tab 0.25 mg, #1/2, P.O., q8h, p.r.n.

         LABORATORY:
            9/11        CBC w/diff 1500 today
            9/11        SMA 27 1500 today
            9/11        SMA 7 0700 tomorrow
            9/11        Sputum C&S/gram stain today

         ANCILLARY:
            9/11        Pulmonary function test at bedside         last page
```

In this computer generated format, information is compact and well-organized.

Use the Kardex to record information that helps nurses plan daily interventions. For example, record the time a patient prefers to bathe, his food preferences before and during chemotherapy, and which analgesics or positions are usually required to ease pain.

The medication Kardex

If your facility uses a separate medication Kardex on acute care units, you'll find this document on the medication cart or other designated place. The medication Kardex may include the medication administration record (MAR), which lists medications, doses, and frequency and route of administration. Medication administration is documented on this form, which is a permanent part of the patient's record. (See *The medication Kardex*, pages 114 and 115.)

Getting the most out of your medication Kardex

When recording information on a medication Kardex, here are some tips:
• Include the date and administration time as well as the medication dose, route, and frequency. Don't forget to initial the entry.
• Indicate when you administer a stat dose of a medication and, if appropriate, the number of doses ordered and the stop date.
• Write legibly, using only standard abbreviations. When in doubt about how to abbreviate a term, spell it out. Remember, the MAR is a legal record, so any information entered there should be legible and above question.
• After giving the first dose of a medication, sign your full name, your licensure status, and your initials in the appropriate space.
• After withholding a medication dose, document which dose wasn't given (usually by circling the time it was scheduled). Also document the reason it was omitted; for example, withholding oral medications from a patient because he has surgery scheduled that day.

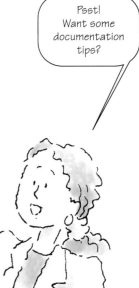

Psst! Want some documentation tips?

Extra, added information

If you administer all medications according to the plan of care, you don't need to document further. However, if your MAR doesn't have space for some information, such as the parenteral administration site, the patient's response to

(Text continues on page 116.)

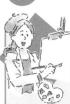

Art of the chart

The medication Kardex

One type of Kardex is the medication Kardex. It contains a permanent record of the patient's medications. The medication Kardex may also include the patient's diagnosis and information about allergies and diet. A sample form is shown below.

NURSE'S FULL SIGNATURE, STATUS AND INITIALS	INIT.		INIT.		INIT.
Roy Charles, RN	RC				
Theresa Hopkins, RN	TH				

Don't forget to sign your name.

DIAGNOSIS: Heart failure, Atrial flutter

ALLERGIES: ASA   **DIET:** Cardiac

ROUTINE/DAILY ORDERS/FINGERSTICKS/ INSULIN COVERAGE	DATE: 11/25/91	DATE:	DATE:	DATE:	DATE:	DATE:	DATE:	DATE:	DATE:	DATE:

ORDER DATE INIT.	RE-NEWAL DATE INIT.	MEDICATIONS DOSE, ROUTE, FREQUENCY	TIME	SITE	INT.	SITE	INT.	SITE	INT.	SITE	INT.	SITE	INT.	SITE	INT.	SITE	INT.	SITE	INT.	SITE	INT.	SITE	INT.
11/24/91		digoxin 0.125 mg	0900	Rs.c	RC																		
RC		I.V. q.d.	HR		TH																		
11/24/91		furosemide 40 mg	0900	Rs.c	RC																		
11/24/91		I.V. q/2h	2100		TH																		
11/24/91		enalapril	0511	Rs.c	TH																		
RC		1.25 mg I.V. q/6h	1100		RC																		
			1700		RC																		
11/25/91		vancomycin 1 g I.V. q.d.	2100	Rs.c	TH																		
TH																							

Initial here to verify that the dose, route, and frequency were checked against the doctor's orders.

The medication Kardex (continued)

	PRN MEDICATION						

Addressograph

ALLERGIES: ASA

INITIAL	SIGNATURE & STATUS	INITIAL	SIGNATURE & STATUS	INITIAL	SIGNATURE & STATUS	INITIAL	SIGNATURE & STATUS
RC	Roy Charles, RN						
TH	Theresa Hopkins, RN						

YEAR 19 _91_   P.R.N. MEDICATIONS

ORDER DATE: 11/24	RENEWAL DATE: /	DISCONTINUED DATE: /	DATE	11/24							
MEDICATION: acetaminophen		DOSE 650 mg	TIME GIVEN	0930							
DIRECTION: p.r.n. mild pain		ROUTE: P.O.	DATA								
			INIT.	RC							

ORDER DATE: 11/24	RENEWAL DATE: /	DISCONTINUED DATE: /	DATE	11/24							
MEDICATION: MSO₄		DOSE 2 mg	TIME GIVEN	0930							
DIRECTION: 15 minutes prior to changing (R) heel dressing		ROUTE: I.V.	DATA								
			INIT.	RC							

ORDER DATE: 11/24	RENEWAL DATE: /	DISCONTINUED DATE: /	DATE	11/24							
MEDICATION: Milk of Magnesia		DOSE 30 ml	TIME GIVEN	2115							
DIRECTION: q6h p.r.n.		ROUTE: P.O.	DATA								
			INIT.	TH							

ORDER DATE: 11/25	RENEWAL DATE: /	DISCONTINUED DATE: 11/25	DATE	11/25							
MEDICATION: prochlorperazine		DOSE 5 mg	TIME GIVEN	1100	2230						
DIRECTION: q6h p.r.n.		ROUTE: I.M.	DATA P.O.	(R) glut.	(L) glut.						
prn nausea and vomiting			INIT.	RC	TH						

ORDER DATE: /	RENEWAL DATE: /	DISCONTINUED DATE: /	DATE								
MEDICATION:		DOSE	TIME GIVEN								
DIRECTION:		ROUTE:	DATA								
			INIT.								

I.M. sites must be charted.

ORDER DATE: /	RENEWAL DATE: /	DISCONTINUED DATE: /	DATE								
MEDICATION:		DOSE	TIME GIVEN								
DIRECTION:		ROUTE:	DATA								
			INIT.								

ORDER DATE: /	RENEWAL DATE: /	DISCONTINUED DATE: /	DATE								
MEDICATION:		DOSE	TIME GIVEN								
DIRECTION:		ROUTE:	DATA								
			INIT.								

p.r.n. medications, or deviations from the medication order, you'll need to record this information in the progress notes. For example, consider the progress note shown below.

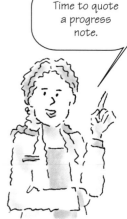

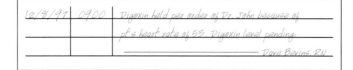

12/8/97	0900	Digoxin held per order of Dr. John because of
		pt's heart rate of 53. Digoxin level pending.
		—————————————————— Dave Bevins, RN

Graphic form

The graphic form is used to plot the patient's vital signs. Weight, intake and output, appetite, and activity level also may be documented on the graphic form. (See *Plotting along: Using a graphic form.*)

The graphic form usually has a column of data printed on the left side of the page, times and dates written across the top, and open blocks within the side and top borders.

Advantages of graphic forms

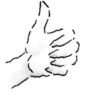

The graphic form has two important advantages:
• They present information at a glance. This allows more visual comparison of data than is possible in narrative-style forms. For example, if a patient's temperature goes up or down or fluctuates over time, this can be detected much more readily on a graph than in a narrative account of the patient's temperatures.
• Unlicensed personnel (such as nursing assistants and technicians) are allowed to document measurements on graphic forms, saving nurses valuable time.

Disadvantages of graphic forms

Guess what. Graphic forms also have disadvantages:
• If data placed on the graph aren't accurate, legible, and complete, the form is useless. Every vital sign you take should be transcribed onto the form. For accuracy, double-check the graph after transcribing information.
• If you use information from the graph alone, you won't get a complete picture of the patient's clinical condition. You must combine the graph with narrative documentation.

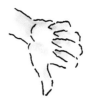

> *Art of the chart*

Plotting along: Using a graphic form

Plotting information on a graphic form helps you visualize changes in your patient's temperature, blood pressure, heart rate, weight, and intake and output. Review the sample form below.

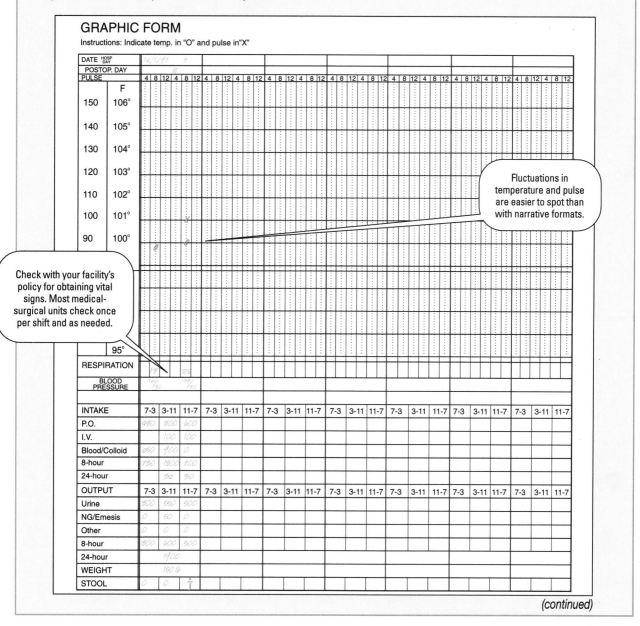

GRAPHIC FORM

Instructions: Indicate temp. in "O" and pulse in "X"

Fluctuations in temperature and pulse are easier to spot than with narrative formats.

Check with your facility's policy for obtaining vital signs. Most medical-surgical units check once per shift and as needed.

(continued)

Plotting along: Using a graphic form (continued)

Additional space is usually provided for more frequently monitored vital signs.

DATE	TIME	BLOOD PRESSURE	PULSE	RESP.	MISCELLANEOUS
12/1/91	0800	130/80	96	20	T 99⁴ blood transfusion
	0815	134/82	102	18	T 99⁸ no s/s of reaction
	0830	128/84	91	16	T 99²

How to use a graphic form

Document directly onto a graphic form when information is obtained, to avoid transcription errors.

A couple more charting opportunities

If a medication (an antipyretic or antihypertensive, for example) precipitates a change in a particular vital sign, document this in the progress notes as well as the graphic form. Specify the relationship between the medication and its effect.

Make sure you also document vital signs on both the graphic form and progress notes when a patient has an acute episode, such as chest pain or a seizure. Be sure to:
• chart legibly
• put data in the correct time line
• make the dots you plot on the graph large enough to be seen easily. (Connect the dots if your facility requires this.)

Progress notes and flow sheets

In the acute care setting, progress notes and flow sheets are used to record the patient's status and monitor changes in his condition.

Making progress with progress notes

Progress notes are written chronologically. The standard format for nursing progress notes has a column for the

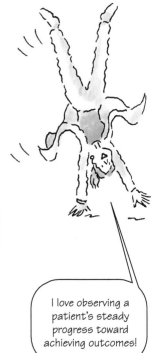

I love observing a patient's steady progress toward achieving outcomes!

date and time and a column for detailed comments about the following:
• the patient's problems (the nursing diagnoses)
• the patient's needs
• pertinent nursing observations
• nursing reassessments and interventions
• the patient's responses to interventions
• progress toward meeting expected outcomes.

Integrated progress notes can be documented by all members of the health care team. This type of note is in chronological order based on the date. (See *A group effort: Integrated progress notes*, page 120.)

Advantages of progress notes

Progress notes are helpful for the following reasons:
• They're written chronologically and reflect the nursing diagnoses.
• They contain narrative information that doesn't easily fit into available space or format provided by other documentation forms.

Disadvantages of progress notes

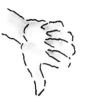

On the other hand, progress notes have these pitfalls:
• If they aren't well organized, you may have to read through the entire form to find what you're looking for. To help prevent this, some facilities require you to put a heading on each note.
• They may contain insignificant information because the documenter feels compelled to fill in space.
• You may waste time recording information on progress notes that you've already recorded on other forms.

Writing clear, accurate progress notes is an art form.

How to write progress notes

When writing progress notes, include the following information:
• date and time of the entry
• the patient's condition
• interventions
• the patient's response to care
• details of changes in the patient's condition
• interventions and their effects.

A group effort: Integrated progress notes

One key advantage of these notes: every member of the health care team can document on them. Integrated progress notes are written in chronological order and dated.

> Don't skip lines between entries.

INTEGRATED PROGRESS NOTES

11/24/91	0800	Nursing note

Pt with temp. 102°F. Doctor Weber notified. No order at this time. ———————————— P. Smith, RN

11/24/91   0830   MICU attending

Pt continues to appear w/o change in status. Remains febrile and unresponsive. Will discuss code status with family. Prognosis poor. ———————————— R. Weber, MD

11/24/91   1030   Infectious disease attending

Pt continues with fever of unknown origin. T max. 104°F. Tylenol ineffective. Cultures from 11/23 pending. Change all central line accesses and send tips for culture. Continue vancomycin, gentamicin, and amikacin. Monitor trough levels and adjust dosages accordingly. Try to obtain HIV testing consent from family. Send fungal cultures. If positive for fungemia, amphotericin B, use test dose. Consult renal for worsening renal failure. ———————————— J. Barry, MD

11/24/91   1545   Intern progress note

HIV consent obtained. Labs to be drawn. ———————————— J. Krimm, DO

> Make sure you record the date and time.

A solid base of nursing diagnoses

Some progress notes are designed to focus on nursing diagnoses. If your facility uses this type of note, be sure to record the nursing diagnosis that relates to your entry. (See *Nursing diagnosis–based progress notes*.)

Set your watch

Every time you write a progress note, be sure to record the exact time you gave the care or noted the observation. Don't record entries in blocks of time, such as 3:30 to 8:30. Years ago, when nurses were required to write progress notes every 2 hours, charting blocks of time was common. But today, most nurses use a flow sheet to chart how often they check on a patient. Together, flow sheets and progress notes usually provide adequate evidence of nursing care.

Change in condition? Chart it.

Be sure to document new patient problems such as *onset of seizures,* and the resolution of old problems such as *no complaint of pain in 12 hours.* Also record deteriorations in the patient's condition; for example, *Pt has increasing dyspnea, causing him to remain on bed rest. ABG values show PaO₂ of 55. O₂ provided by rebreather mask as ordered.*

Document your observations of the patient's response to the plan of care. If his behaviors are similar to agreed-upon objectives, document that the goals are being met. If not, document that they aren't being met.

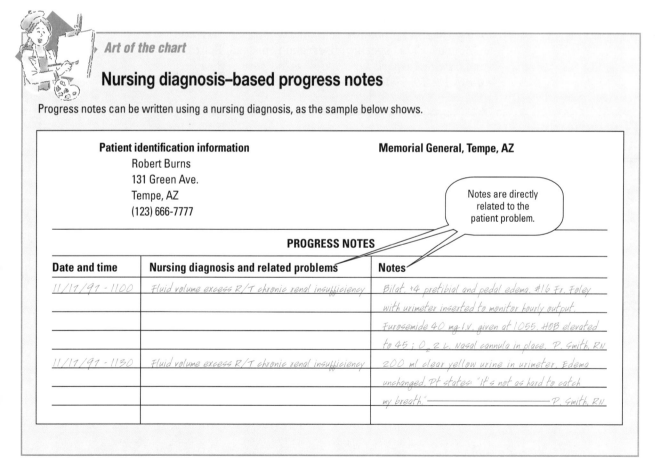

Art of the chart

Nursing diagnosis–based progress notes

Progress notes can be written using a nursing diagnosis, as the sample below shows.

Patient identification information
Robert Burns
131 Green Ave.
Tempe, AZ
(123) 666-7777

Memorial General, Tempe, AZ

Notes are directly related to the patient problem.

PROGRESS NOTES

Date and time	Nursing diagnosis and related problems	Notes
11/17/91 - 1100	Fluid volume excess R/T chronic renal insufficiency	Bilat. +4 pretibial and pedal edema. #16 Fr. Foley with urimeter inserted to monitor hourly output. Furosemide 40 mg I.V. given at 1055. HOB elevated to 45°; O₂ 2 L. Nasal cannula in place. P. Smith, RN
11/17/91 - 1130	Fluid volume excess R/T chronic renal insufficiency	200 ml clear yellow urine in urimeter. Edema unchanged. Pt states: "It's not as hard to catch my breath." ———————— P. Smith, RN

Don't repeat yourself

Avoid including information that's already on the flow sheet, except when there's a sudden change in the patient's condition, such as a decreased level of consciousness, change in skin condition, or swelling at an I.V. site.

Say what you did

Sometimes, nurses document a problem but fail to describe what they did about it. Outline your interventions clearly, including such information as notification of other health team members, interventions, and the patient's response. For example, *Patient at 8 a.m. had oral temp of 102° F, Dr. Bard notified. Acetaminophen 650 mg given P.O. At 10 a.m. patient had oral temp. of 100° F.*

Avoid vague wording. Using a phrase like "appears to be" indicates uncertainty about what you're charting. Phrases like "no problems" and "had a good day" are also ambiguous. Chart specific observations instead. For example, *Patient reports his left hip has less pain, a 2 on a scale of 1 to 10. Yesterday it was a 5.*

Flow sheets

Flow sheets highlight specific patient information according to preestablished parameters of nursing care. They have spaces for recording dates, times, and specific interventions.

Charting with a nice flow

Flow sheets are used for charting data related to physical assessment of the patient and for recording routine aspects of patient care, such as activities of daily living, fluid balance, nutrition, pain, and skin integrity. They're also useful for recording specific nursing interventions.

Many facilities also document I.V. therapy and patient education on flow sheets. The style and format of flow sheets may be varied to fit the needs of patients on particular units. Using flow sheets doesn't exempt you from narrative charting to describe your observations, patient teaching, patient responses, detailed interventions, and unusual circumstances. (See *Go with the flow sheets*.)

Art of the chart

Go with the flow sheets

As this sample shows, a patient care flow sheet lets you quickly document routine interventions.

PATIENT CARE FLOW SHEET

Date: 11/22/91	2300-0700	0700-1500	
RESPIRATORY			
Breath sounds	Clear 2330 AS	Crackles LLL 0800 JM	Clear 1600 HM
Treatments/Results	————————	Nebulizer 0830 JM	
Cough/Results	AS	Mod. amt. tenacious yellow mucus 0900 JM	HM
O₂ therapy	Nasal cannula @2 L/min AS	Nasal cannula @2 L/min JM	Nasal cannula @2 L/min HM
CARDIAC			
Chest pain	AS	JM	HM
Heart sounds	Normal S₁ and S₂ AS	Normal S₁ and S₂ JM	Normal S₁ and S₂ HM
Telemetry	N/A	N/A	N/A
PAIN			
Type and location	(L) flank 0400 AS	(L) flank 1000 JM	(L) flank 1600 HM
Intervention	meperidine 0415 AS	reposition and meperidine 1010 JM	meperidine 1615 HM
Pt response	Improved from #9 to #3 in 1/2 hour AS	Improved from #8 to #2 in 1/2 hr JM	complete relief in 1 hr HM
NUTRITION			
Type	————————	regular JM	Regular HM
Toleration %	————————	90% JM	80% HM
Supplement	————————	1 can Ensure JM	————————
ELIMINATION			
Stool appearance	AS	JM	1 HM
Enema	N/A	N/A	N/A
Results	————————	————————	————————
Bowel sounds	present all quadrants 2330 AS	present all quadrants 0800 JM	hyperactive all quadrants 1600 HM
Urine appearance	clear amber 0400 AS	clear amber 1000 JM	Dark yellow 1500 HM
Indwelling urinary catheter	N/A	N/A	N/A
Catheter irrigations	————————		————————

Callouts:

Be sure to initial your entry.

Note the exact time.

Make sure you document your patient's response to medications.

Use the flow sheet to track changes in your patient's responses.

(continued)

Go with the flow sheets *(continued)*

PATIENT CARE FLOW SHEET

Date 11/22/91	2300-0700	0700-1500	1500-2300
TUBES			
Type	N/A	N/A	N/A
Irrigation			
Drainage appearance			
HYGIENE			
Self/partial/ complete		Partial 1000 JM	Partial 2100 HM
Oral care		1000 JM	2100 HM
Back care	0400 AS	1000 JM	2100 HM
Foot care		1000 JM	
Remove/reapply elastic stockings	2330 AS	1000 JM	2100 HM
ACTIVITY			
Type	bed rest AS	OOB to chair x 20 min 1000 JM	OOB to chair x 20 min 1800 HM
Toleration	Turns self AS	Tol. well JM	Tol. well
Repositioned	2330 supine AS 0400 (L) side AS	(L) side 0800 JM (R) side 1400 JM	self HM
ROM		1000 (active) JM 1400 (active) JM	1800 (active) HM 2200 (active) HM
SLEEP			
Sleeps well	0400 AS 0600 AS	N/A	N/A
Awake at intervals	2300 AS 0400 AS		
Awake most of the time			
SAFETY			
ID bracelet on	2330 AS 0200 AS	0800 JM 1200 JM 1500 JM	1600 HM 2100 HM
Call button in reach	2330 AS 0200 AS	0800 JM 1200 JM 1500 JM	1600 HM 2100 HM
Side rails up	2330 AS 0200 AS	0800 JM 1200 JM 1500 JM	1600 HM 2100 HM

Don't leave space blank. Write "none" or "N/A" or draw a line through the space.

Flow sheets encourage you to chart care promptly.

Advantages of flow sheets

Flow sheets have many sterling qualities. For example:
• You can insert nursing data quickly and concisely, preferably at the time you give care or observe a change in the patient's condition.
• Because they provide an easy-to-read record of changes in the patient's condition over time, flow sheets allow all members of the health care team to compare data and assess the patient's progress.
• The concise format enables you to evaluate patient trends at a glance.
• They're less time-consuming to read because they tend to be more legible than completely handwritten progress notes.
• The format reinforces standards of nursing care and facilitates precise and less-fragmented nursing documentation. This makes the information more useful to the health care team and more helpful to defense lawyers, if the need arises.

> Flow sheets are easy to prepare and easy to read!

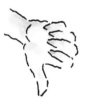

Disadvantages of flow sheets

Flow sheets also have some less-than-ideal qualities. For example:
• They don't have enough space for recording unusual events.
• Overuse of these forms can lead to incomplete documentation that obscures the patient's clinical picture.
• They may cause legal hassles if they're not consistent with the progress notes. This can occur if you hurriedly check off whatever the previous nurse checked off, and then chart the actual care on the progress notes.
• The format may fail to reflect the patients' needs and the nurses' documentation needs on each unit. Flow sheets can become a liability if they don't reflect these needs or aren't revised as needs change.
• They add bulk to the medical record, causing handling and storage problems and duplication of documentation.

How to use flow sheets

Ideally, flow sheets are used to document all routine assessment data and nursing interventions. Some common examples of these are:
• repositioning or turning the patient
• range-of-motion exercises
• patient education

- wound care
- medication administration.

Charting routine assessment data this way allows you to focus on changes in the patient's condition, his complex needs, and his progress toward achieving expected outcomes.

Be sure data on the flow sheet are consistent with data in your progress notes. Of course, all entries should accurately reflect the care given. Discrepancies can damage your credibility and increase your chance of liability.

Completing the picture

Sometimes, recording only the information requested isn't enough to give a complete picture of the patient's health. If this is the case, record additional information in the space provided on the flow sheet. If additional information isn't necessary, draw a line through the space to indicate this.

If your flow sheet doesn't have additional space and you need to record more information, use the progress notes.

Symbolic significance

Fill out flow sheets completely, using the specified symbols — such as check marks, Xs, initials, circles, or the time — to indicate assessment of a parameter or performance of an intervention. When necessary, use the abbreviation "N/A" (not applicable) or another abbreviation recognized by your facility.

Ban the blanks

Don't leave blank spaces, which may imply that an intervention either wasn't completed, wasn't attempted, or wasn't recognized. If you must omit something, document the reason for the omission.

Discharge summaries

Discharge summaries reflect the reassessment and evaluation components of the nursing process. To comply with JCAHO requirements, you must document your assessment of a patient's continuing care needs as well as any referrals for care.

Before we say goodbye...

To help in this kind of documentation, many facilities combine discharge summaries and patient instructions in

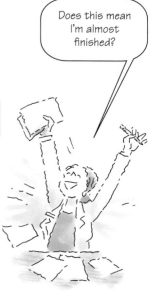

Does this mean I'm almost finished?

one form. This form contains sections for recording patient assessment, patient education, detailed special instructions, and the circumstances of discharge. It uses a narrative style along with open- and close-ended styles. (See *Moving on: Discharge summaries.*)

Art of the chart

Moving on: Discharge summaries

By combining the patient's discharge summary with instructions for care after discharge, you can fulfill two requirements with a single form. When using this documentation method, be sure to give one copy to the patient and keep one for the record.

DISCHARGE INSTRUCTIONS

1. SUMMARY *Tara Nicholas is a 55 year old woman admitted with complaints of severe headache and hypertensive crisis.*

Treatment: Nipride gtt for 24 hours

Started Lopressor for hypertension

Recommendation: Lose 10-15 lbs

Follow low Na, low cholesterol diet

> Have the patient or a family member read the medication instruction back to you.

2. ALLERGIES *penicillin*

3. MEDICATIONS (drug, dose time) *Lopressor 25 mg at 6am and 6pm*

temazepam 15 mg at 10pm

> Write instructions clearly so the patient or family can easily understand them. This is the form they'll refer to when they're trying to remember your teaching.

4. DIET *Low sodium, low cholesterol*

5. ACTIVITY *As tolerated*

6. DISCHARGED TO *Home*

7. IF QUESTIONS ARISE, CONTACT DR. *Pritchett*   TELEPHONE NO. *525-1448*

8. SPECIAL INSTRUCTIONS

9. RETURN VISIT DR. *Pritchett*   PLACE *Health Care Clinic*

ON DATE *12/15/91*   TIME *8:45 am*

Tara Nicholas   *JE PRITCHETT MD*

| SIGNATURE OF PATIENT FOR RECEIPT OF INSTRUCTIONS FROM DOCTORS | SIGNATURE OF DOCTOR GIVING INSTRUCTIONS |

Advantages of discharge summaries

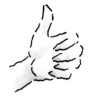

We have only good things to say about discharge summary forms:

• The combined form provides useful data about additional teaching needs and points out whether the patient has the information he needs to care for himself or to get further help.

• The form establishes compliance with JCAHO requirements and helps safeguard you from malpractice accusations.

How to use discharge summaries

After completing your discharge summary, give one copy of the form to the patient and put another copy in the medical record for future reference. Be sure that the completed form outlines the patient's care, provides useful information for further teaching and evaluation, and documents that the patient has the information he needs to care for himself or to get further help.

Taking note of narrative discharge notes

Not all facilities use combined forms — some use narrative discharge summaries. (See *Parting words: Narrative discharge notes.*) If your facility uses these, be sure to include the following information on the form:

Art of the chart

Parting words: Narrative discharge notes

Some health care facilities use a narrative-style discharge summary, which is similar to a progress note. Here's a sample:

Date	Time	Progress notes
12/1/91	Discharge 1530 (summary)	68 y.o. black male admitted 11/28/91 with chest pain, hypertension; BP 190/100, and SOB. MI ruled out. Chest pain relieved with sublingual nitroglycerin and O₂. Persantine thallium performed 11/30. Tolerated procedure well. Has been OOB ambulating in the hallway without chest pain or SOB since 11/30. BP remains stable (144/86 at 1215). Drug regimen includes daily aspirin 325 mg, and Captopril 25 mg b.id. Verbalized understanding of medication times, dosages, and adverse effects. Will call Dr. Harris for 10 day postdischarge appointment. Discharge instruction sheet given.——— B. McCort, RN

• the patient's status at admission and discharge
• significant information about the patient's stay in the facility, including resolved and unresolved patient problems and referrals for continuing care
• instructions given to the patient, members of his family, and other caregivers about medications, treatments, activity, diet, referrals, follow-up appointments, and any other special instructions.

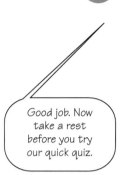

Good job. Now take a rest before you try our quick quiz.

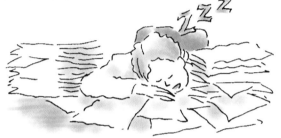

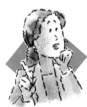

Quick quiz

1. An admission database is:
   A. a collection of computer information about your patient's psychosocial status.
   B. a form that documents your initial patient assessment data.
   C. a collection of data printed by a computer.

Answer: B. It's also known as an admission assessment form.

2. Which of the following is a responsibility of the staff nurse in the discharge planning process?
   A. initiating a referral for home health services
   B. evaluating the patient's mental status when his competence is an issue
   C. deciding when the patient should be discharged

Answer: A. Initiating a referral for home health services is within the nurse's scope of practice.

3. A care track is an important part of:
   A. a computer-generated Kardex.
   B. a critical pathway.
   C. a flow sheet.

Answer: B. The care track, or case map, defines a patient's daily care requirements and desired outcomes, consistent with the average length of stay for a specified DRG.

4. Progress notes are organized by:
    A. alphabetical order.
    B. numerical order.
    C. chronological order.

Answer: C. Progress notes chronologically record the patient's status and track changes in his condition.

5. The JCAHO asks nurses to do all of the following except:
    A. include a patient care Kardex in the medical record.
    B. include ongoing assessments related to illness in plans of care.
    C. use flow sheets to document basic assessment findings and wound care, hygiene, and routine care interventions.

Answer: A. A Kardex isn't a JCAHO requirement, so some facilities have eliminated it and incorporated the information into the patient's plan of care. Answer B is a JCAHO requirement; answer C is a request.

Scoring

☆☆☆   If you answered all five items correctly, amazing! You're destined to be acclaimed for accurate observation of acute care.

☆☆   If you answered three or four correctly, wonderful! Your progress is well-noted.

☆   If you answered fewer than three correctly, don't worry. You can take the test as many times as you want and record your scores on a flow sheet.

Home health care

In this chapter, you'll learn:

◆ current trends in home health care

◆ risks and responsibilities in documenting home health care

◆ forms used for home health care documentation

◆ documenting patient teaching in home health care

◆ future trends in home health care.

A look at home health care

The purpose of home health nursing is to restore, maintain, or promote health for patients and their families at home. A home health agency plans, coordinates, and supplies care based on the needs of the patient and family and the resources available to them. Think of the home health agency as a hospital without walls. Home care is one component of comprehensive health care.

An emerging health care powerhouse

Recent trends have contributed to the growth of the home health care industry:

• the development of the national system of diagnosis-related groups (DRGs)

• the increasing number of managed care organizations competing for health care dollars

• the increasing number of patients of all ages

• increased availability of safe, easily operated health care equipment.

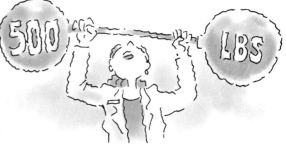

Get me to the home health agency on time

DRGs are used to predetermine Medicare reimbursement to health care facilities based on patients' medical diagnoses and anticipated lengths of stay. Under this system, a facility that discharges a patient to be cared for at home before his maximum length of stay is up increases its profit margin. The use of DRGs has increased pressure for on-time discharge of patients from hospitals.

Strength in diversity

Managed care organizations are becoming increasingly severe with regard to limiting hospital admissions and length of stay. In response, hospitals are diversifying outpatient services and establishing integrated delivery systems. Integrated delivery systems usually include home health care agencies.

Because support services in the home and community cost less than institutional care, government and private insurance payers are expanding their coverage of home health care. In the future, the home health industry may become the primary supplier of health care in the United States.

Not your traditional patient

Traditionally, homebound Medicare recipients have constituted the major portion of the home health caseload. Now, agencies are expanding services to new populations, representing all age groups and a variety of medical conditions. This has led to the emergence of home health subspecialties such as home infusion agencies. These agencies may be offshoots of parent organizations or stand-alone agencies. (See *The hospice alternative.*)

Guess what. New documentation requirements

Because an increasing number of people covered by private insurance plans receive home care, agencies have had to adapt to the documentation and billing requirements of many different third-party payers. These requirements differ substantially from the Medicare guidelines, forms, and requirements with which agencies are familiar.

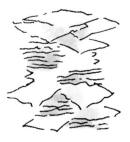

The hospice alternative

Many home health care agencies provide hospice care services. Hospice programs provide palliative care to the terminally ill in both home and hospital.

Medicare coverage

Since 1983, patients who have met specific admission criteria can qualify for the hospice Medicare benefit instead of the traditional Medicare benefit, allowing greater freedom to choose the hospice alternative for terminal care. The patient receives noncurative medical and support service not otherwise covered by Medicare.

Medicare coverage for hospice care is available if:

• The patient is eligible for Medicare Part A which covers skilled nursing home and hospital care. People eligible for Medicare are those age 65 or older, the long-term disabled, and people with end-stage renal disease.

• The patient's doctor and the hospice medical director certify that the patient is terminally ill with a life expectancy of six months or less.

• The patient receives care from a Medicare-approved hospice program.

A Medicare-approved hospice will usually provide care in the patient's home. The hospice and the patient's doctor establish a plan of care for medical and support services for the management of a terminal illness.

A patient without coverage for hospice benefits may be eligible for free or reduced cost care through local programs or foundations. Alternatively, a patient may pay privately for hospice services.

Understanding and acceptance of treatment

With hospice care, the patient and primary caregiver must complete documentation indicating their understanding of hospice care. The patient and caregiver must sign an informed consent form that outlines everyone's responsibilities. The patient and primary caregiver must also sign a form indicating understanding and acceptance of the role of the primary caregiver. The form below is an example of this type of document.

REEDSVILLE HOME HEALTH AND HOSPICE
ACCEPTANCE OF PRIMARY CAREGIVER ROLE

I have been offered the opportunity to ask questions regarding the Hospice program and Hospice care of this patient. I understand that the Hospice program provides palliative, or comfort measures and services, but not aggressive, invasive, or life sustaining procedures.

I also understand that the Hospice concept of care is based upon the active participation of a primary care person who is not provided through the Hospice benefit, who is and will be willing to assist this patient with personal care and with activities of daily living as well as with safety precautions when Hospice personnel are not scheduled to be in the home. I accept the responsibility of being primary caregiver, and I agree to make appropriate arrangements to provide this role to this patient.

If, for any reason, I am unable to serve in this capacity at a time as deemed necessary for the safety and care of this patient, I agree to make other arrangements to fulfill the responsibilities of primary caregiver, which are acceptable to Reedsville Home Health and Hospice. I further understand that Reedsville Home Health and Hospice will assist in making the arrangements, but that I will be financially responsible for any costs associated with them.

Name of Patient: _Joan Powell_

Signature of Patient: _Joan Powell_

Date: _11/17/91_

Name of primary caregiver: _Joseph Powell_

Date: _11/17/91_

Signature of primary caregiver: _Joseph Powell_

Relationship: _husband_

Witness: _Cathy Melvin, RN_

Date: _11/17/91_

> When the patient and caregiver sign this form, it indicates that they understand the purpose and goals of hospice care.

Creating opportunities for care

Before receiving care from a home health care agency, most patients must obtain authorization from their insurance provider. In many cases, insurance limitations restrict treatment options. In this cost-conscious environment, nurses can take on an especially important role in helping patients get coverage by educating them about local, state, and federal benefit programs. When you help a patient identify a program for which he qualifies — such as veteran's benefits or Meals on Wheels — you help him get the services he needs while ensuring that your agency receives proper reimbursement.

Legal risks and responsibilities

Home health agencies are licensed and regulated by state governments and accredited by private agencies such as the Community Health Accreditation Program (CHAP), which is administered through the National League for Nursing (NLN) and the Joint Commission on Accreditation of Healthcare Organizations (JCAHO). In many cases, obtaining state licensure hinges on having accreditation. Home health agencies must also adhere to Medicare and Medicaid regulations administered by the Health Care Financing Administration (HCFA) and its agencies and carriers.

Home health agencies are evaluated for such factors as accurate and complete documentation, adherence to standards, and quality of care. If standards aren't met, a home health agency may fail to earn licensure or accreditation, have its current license and accreditation revoked, or have reimbursement privileges withheld or revoked.

Looking it up

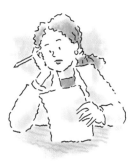

All state boards of nursing require home health agencies to maintain updated nursing policy and procedure manuals and to make them available to staff. Policy and procedure manuals cover such key nursing issues as documentation, nursing procedures, patient education, patient health progress, and patient compliance.

The home health agency's policies and procedures manual is the final word on your responsibilities in professional home health care practice. Nursing management should review and update manuals annually (more frequently, if necessary) and have all policies and procedures signed and dated by each employee.

Risks of poor documentation

Home health agencies must maintain complete and legally sound documentation. For reimbursable services, nurses must document each instance that the specified service is provided. Nurses must also document the services the agency refuses to provide. Inadequate or incomplete documentation can have serious consequences.

Inappropriate care

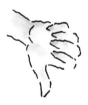

Cursory care plans that don't fully reflect the patient's needs and resources may result in incomplete or inappropriate care. For example, a visually impaired diabetic patient is taught to self-administer insulin, but his care plan does not include evaluation and teaching of foot care. Such a patient is at risk for serious foot problems, including amputations.

The fact that family members or friends commonly act as caregivers to home health patients makes accurate documentation even more vital. For example, a tired home health care nurse administers a potent pain medication but forgets to document it or mention it to the patient's husband, who is caregiver for the next shift. The patient's husband gives another dose of medication shortly after the nurse leaves. Because of the communication gap, the patient could go into respiratory arrest.

Liability

Once a nurse or home health agency is named in a lawsuit, it's too late to correct inaccurate documentation. For example, a nurse fails to record the patient's apical pulse and rhythm before administering digoxin. Later, the family sues the home health agency, alleging the staff caused the patient to go into complete heart block by failing to recognize signs of digitalis toxicity. Without a documented record, the agency is unable to prove that the patient wasn't experiencing excessive slowing of the pulse, a classic sign of digitalis toxicity.

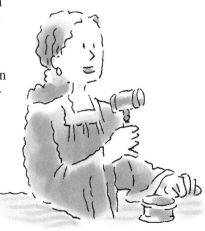

Financial losses

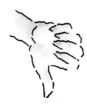

Inadequate or incomplete documentation may result in third-party payers refusing to cover services. In addition to harming the agency, this may cause the patient to pay unexpected out-of-pocket expenses that otherwise would have been reimbursed.

Insurance companies who negotiate preferred provider contracts may refuse to do business with home health agencies that provide shoddy documentation; plenty of competing agencies will willingly provide excellent documentation along with comparable services.

Does the patient qualify?

Careful screening, which is done at the initial evaluation, is critical when determining what clinical services a patient needs. When evaluating a new patient for service, look for the following criteria:

Clinical criteria
• Medically stable condition
• Appropriately prescribed therapy
• Appropriate diagnosis
• Appropriate vascular access device, if needed

Technical criteria
• Visual ability
• Manual dexterity
• Capability of learning and following procedures
• Capability of recognizing complications and initiating emergency medical procedures

Environmental criteria
• Access to a telephone
• Access to electricity
• Access to water
• Clean living environment

Financial criteria
• Verification of insurance coverage
• Full knowledge of co-payment or out-of-pocket expenses

> My patient's care depends on my astute evaluation of his need for services.

Documentation guidelines

Documentation of care and discharge planning begins when you evaluate a new patient for service. (See *Does the patient qualify?*) You may use a referral form to document the patient's needs. (See *Referral form*, pages 138 and 139.) Patients and caregivers also fill out several forms during the initial home visit. (See *Paperwork for patients.*)

Once you start caring for a patient, always document activities completed during your nursing visit: assessments, interventions, the patient's response to treatment, and whether he had complications. Also record your communications with other members of the health care team and the date of the next visit. Consider using flow sheets to document routine nursing care.

Love to do the "utilization review"

The information you provide is used by third-party payers during utilization review to evaluate each claim in accordance with criteria for coverage.

Six (count 'em) points

Home care documentation should cover the following items:
• evidence that the home environment is safe for the procedure or treatment or can be safely adapted; findings about the home and measures taken to ensure safe delivery of care
• rationale for treatment and patient response
• emergency and resource numbers given to patient or caregiver (JCAHO requires that the patient or caregiver have 24-hour emergency telephone access to the agency or nurse.)
• the patient's or caregiver's ability to perform steps in home care procedures, including the patient's or caregiver's ability to perform return demonstration
• The patient's or caregiver's ability to troubleshoot equipment, including a backup plan for a power failure
• the patient's or caregiver's ability to recognize potential complications, respond appropriately, and get help when necessary.

Paperwork for patients

During your initial home visit, you'll ask the patient or caregiver to read and sign many forms. These required forms include the following:
• patient rights and responsibilities
• advance directives, including a do-not-resuscitate option
• consent for services
• medical information authorization and release
• assignment of benefits
• equipment acceptance
• patient-teaching checklist.

If an I.V. infusion is required, the forms also include:
• consent for vascular access
• infusion treatment service agreement.

Documenting patient teaching

Correct documentation will help justify to your agency and to third-party payers your visits to teach the patient or caregiver. Find out about the patient's and family's needs,

(Text continues on page 140.)

Art of the chart

Referral form

Also called an intake form, this form is used to document the patient's needs when you begin your evaluation of a new patient. Use the form below as a guide.

Date of referral: *11/17/91*   Branch   *North*

> This form provides an overview of the patient's condition, required treatment, and psychosocial and cultural concerns.

Chart #: *97-413*   H ✓

Info taken by: *Beth Isham, RN   North*   Admit Date: *11/18/91*

Patient's Name: *Geraldine Rush*

Address: *66 Newton St.*

City: *Burlington*   *VT*   Zip: *05402*

Phone: *(802) 123-4561*   Date of birth: *4/3/20*

Primary caregiver name & phone number: *husband (Dennis) (802) 123-4561*

Insurance name: *Medicare*   Ins. #: *123-45-6189*

Is this a managed care policy (HMO)? *no*

Primary Dx: (Code *162.5*)   *lung cancer*   Date: *12/11/96*

(Code *811*)   *decubitus ulcer (coccyx)*   Date: *3/13/91*

(Code *714.0*)   *rheumatoid arthritis*   Date: *1980s*

Procedures: (Code *86.28*)   *decubitus care*   Date: *11/1/91*

Referral source: *J. Silva, hospital SW*   Phone: *165-2813*

Doctor name & phone #: *Frank Crabbe*   Phone: *165-4321*

Doctor address: *9013 Parkway Drive, Burlington*

Hospital *university Hospital*   Admit *11/1/91*   Discharge *11/16/91*

Functional limitations: Pain management, *nonambulatory, poor fine motor skills 2° rheum*

ORDERS/SERVICES: (specify amount, frequency and duration)

> Check out this part of the form to determine what services the patient needs.

(SN:) *SN visits 3x/week & p.r.n. x 2 months*

(AL:) *CNA visits daily 5 days/week x 2 months*

(PT, OT,)ST: *PT & OT evaluations and visits 2-3 x/week & p.r.n. x 2 month*

(MSW:) *MSW evaluation & weekly vs x 2 months*

Spiritual Coordinator: *Rev. Carlson, St. Paul's Lutheran Church*

Counselor: *JoAnne Knowlton, MSW*

Volunteer: *Rosalie Marshall - niece will provide care on weekends*

Other services provided: *shopping, laundry, meal prep*

Goals: *wound care, pain management, terminal care @ home*

Equipment: *needs: commode, hospital bed, bedpan, Hoyer lift, side rail w/c*

Company & Phone number: *Scott Medical Equipment 165-9931*

Safety Measures *side rails*   Nutritional req *diet as tolerated*

FUNCTIONAL LIMITATIONS: (Circle Applicable)			ACTIVITIES PERMITTED: (Circle Applicable)		
1 Amputation	5 Paralysis	9 Legally Blind	1. Complete bedrest	6. Partial wgt bearing	A. Wheelchair
2 Bowel/Bladder	6 Endurance	A Dyspnea with	2. Bedrest BRP	7. Independent at home	B. Walker
3 Contracture	7 Ambulation	minimal exer	3. Up as tolerated	8. Crutches	C. No restriction
4 Hearing	8 Speech	B. Other *R.A.*	4. Transfer bed/chair	9. Cane	D. Other -specify

Accessibility to bath Y - N   Shower Y - N   Bathroom Y - N   Exit Y - N

Mental status: (Circle) Oriented Comatose Forgetful Depressed Disoriented Lethargic Agitated Other

Referral form (continued)

Allergies: _____none known_____

- Hospice appropriate meds
  - MEDICATIONS:

• Med company: _____Walker Pharmacy_____

_____morphine sulfate liq. 20 mg/ml 40 mg P.O. q6h p.r.n. pain_____

_____Compazine 10 mg P.O. or P.R. q4-6h p.r.n. n/v_____

_____Colace 200 mg P.O. q.d. p.r.n. constipation_____

_____Benadryl 25 - 50 mg P.O. @ h.s. p.r.n. sleeplessness_____

Living will   yes ✔   no_____   obtained _____   Family to mail to office _____

Guardian, POA, or responsible person: _____husband_____

Address & phone number: _____same_____

Other family members: _____

ETOH _____0_____ Drug Use: _____0_____ Smoker _2 ppd x 40 years quit 2 yrs ago_

History: _____other than problems associated with arthritis, was in general good health until 12/96, Dx: lung CA - husband cared for_

_____@ home until 11/1/97._

Social history (place of birth, education, jobs, retirement, etc.) _Born & raised in Toronto, became U.S. citizen_

_____when married in 1951. 2 yrs. college - majored in music. Retired church organist._

ADMISSION NOTES: VS: T_98°P.O._   AP _86_   RR _18_   BP _140/72_

Lungs: _breath sounds LLL._   Extremities: _cool to touch Pedal pulses present._

Wgt: _118_ Recent wgt (loss)/gain of _40 lb over 6 months_

Admission narrative: _visit made to pt/husband in hospital before discharge. Both have been told that she is failing rapidly, and_

_____would like her to return home with Hospice services. Niece willing to help 2 days/week. Pt apprehensive; husband blames him_

_____self for the coccygeal decubitus which developed under his care._

Psychosocial Issues _Pt has always cared for husband. Describes self as depressed that she is no longer able to do so;_

_____worries who will care for him after she dies._

Environmental concerns _(need smoke detectors)_

Are there any cultural or spiritual customs or beliefs of which we should be aware before providing

Hospice services? _Pt would like Holy Communion just before death (& weekly)_

Funeral home: _not yet chosen_ Contact made yes_____ no _x_

DIRECTIONS: _corner Newton / Elm   duplex, white with green trim. Door on (L) says 66. Bell broken - knock loudly._

Agency Representative Signature: _Beth Isham, RN_   Date: _11/18/97_

Home Care Supervisor

resources, and support systems. This will help you outline the basic plan for teaching.

Continuity is key

Remember that teaching is usually an ongoing process requiring more than one visit. Until the patient becomes independent, your documentation will help other nurses continue the teaching and identify additional areas of teaching. (See *Certification of instruction*.)

Keep a list of teaching and reference materials you have supplied to the patient or caregiver. Also document modifications made to accommodate the patient's or caregiver's literacy skills and native language.

Be careful and caring...

If the patient isn't physically or mentally able to perform the skills himself and no caregiver is available, report this in your documentation. Never leave a patient alone to perform a procedure until he can express understanding of it and perform it competently.

...and clear and consistent

Be careful to call equipment by the same names used on the packages and in teaching literature. Consider providing a glossary of terms. Make sure that the patient can identify devices when speaking on the telephone. Document all teaching materials given to the patient and keep copies of teaching materials in your records.

Most agencies require patients to sign a teaching documentation record indicating that they accept responsibility for learning self-care activities. This is a critical piece of documentation for the home care chart.

Forms, forms, forms

Key forms used to document home health care include the following:
- agency assessment form
- plan of care
- progress notes
- nursing and discharge summaries.

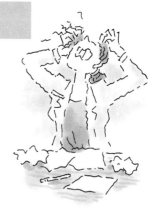

▶ *Art of the chart*

Certification of instruction

The model patient-teaching form below shows what was taught to a home-care patient with an I.V. This type of form will help you document your teaching sessions clearly and completely.

This document helps ensure continuity of patient teaching.

CONTENT (check all that apply; fill in blanks as indicated)

1. ☐ Reason for therapy

2. Drug/Solution
   - ☐ Dose
   - ☐ Schedule
   - ☐ Label accuracy
   - ☐ Storage
   - ☐ Container integrity

3. Aseptic technique
   - ☐ Handwashing
   - ☐ Prepping caps/connections
   - ☐ Tubing/cap/needs
   - ☐ Needless adaptor changes

4. Access device maintenance
   - Type/Name: _____
   - ☒ Device / Site Inspection
   - ☐ Site care/Dsg. changes
   - ☐ Catheter clamping
   - ☒ Maintaining patency
     - ☒ Saline flushing
     - ☐ Heparin locking
     - ☐ Fdg. Tube /declogging
     - ☐ Self insertion of device

5. Drug preparation
   - ☒ Premixed containers
   - ☐ Compounding   ☐ Client additives
   - ☐ Piggyback lipids

6. Method of administration
   - ☐ Gravity
   - ☒ Pump (name): *IVAC pump*
   - ☐ Continuous   ☒ Intermittent
   - ☐ Cycle/Taper:

7. Administration technique
   - ☒ Pump rate/calibration
   - ☐ Priming tubing   ☐ Filter
   - ☐ Filling syringe
   - ☐ Loading pump
   - ☒ Access device hookup/disconnect

8. Potential complications/Adverse effects
   - ☐ Patient drug information sheet reviewed__
   - ☒ Pump alarms/troubleshooting
   - ☒ Phlebitis/infiltration
   - ☐ Clotting/dislodgment
   - ☒ Infection   ☐ Air embolus
   - ☐ Breakage/cracking
   - ☐ Electrolyte imbalance
   - ☐ Fluid balance
   - ☐ Glucose intolerance
   - ☐ Aspiration
   - ☐ N / V / D / Cramping
   - ☐ Other: _____

9. Self monitoring:
   - ☐ Weight   ☒ Temperature   ☐ P   ☐ PB
   - ☐ Urine S & A   ☐ Fingersticks
   - ☐ Other: _____

10. Supply handling/disposal
    - ☒ Disposal of sharps/supplies ☐ Narcotics
    - ☐ Cleaning pump
    - ☒ Changing batteries
    - ☐ Blood/fluid precautions
    - ☐ Chemo/spill precautions

11. Information given to client re:
    - ☐ Pharmacy counseling
    - ☐ Advance directives
    - ☐ Inventory checks _____
    - ☐ Deliveries _____
    - ☒ 24-hour on-call staff _____
    - ☒ Reimbursement_____
    - ☐ Service complaints _____

12. Safety/Disaster plan
    - ☐ Back up pump batteries _____
    - ☒ Emergency room use _____
    - ☒ Electrical _____
    - ☒ Disaster _____
    - ☐ Other: _____

13. Written instructions
    - ☒ Yes ☐ No   If no why _____

☐ Client or caregiver demonstrates or verbalizes competency to perform home infusion therapy.

COMMENTS: _*Wife incorrectly changed pump battery. Procedure reviewed. Wife then demonstrated correct procedure. Wife also concerned about frequency of dressing changes. Access site nonreddened and not edematous. Protocol reviewed patient states he is satisfied to wait until scheduled dressing change tomorrow.*_

The form provides room to comment and to document individual instructions.

Theory/Skill reviewed/Return demonstration completed:

Chris Banner, RN   11-21-91

Signature of RN Educator   **Date**

CERTIFICATION OF INSTRUCTION

I agree that I have been instructed as described above and understand that the above functions will be performed in the home by myself and caregiver, outside a hospital or medically supervised environment.

Robert Burns   11-21-91

Client/caregiver signature   **Date**

In this part of the form, the patient acknowledges responsibility for self-care activities.

Agency assessment form

Once a patient is referred to your home health care agency, you must complete a thorough and specific assessment and chart the information on a patient assessment form. Assess the patient's:
• physical status
• mental and emotional status
• home environment in relation to safety and support services
• knowledge of his disease or current condition, prognosis, and treatment plan
• potential for complying with the treatment plan.

Guidelines for use

As with any setting, be thorough. A thorough patient assessment provides the information you need to plan appropriate care. Consider the following:
• If you are obtaining a health history, obtain information about the patient's past and current health. Organize the interview by body system and ask open-ended questions.
• When taking a physical assessment, use a systematic approach, as is appropriate in any setting. For example, you may take a body-system or head-to-toe approach.
• When assessing the home environment consider such factors as the presence of a caregiver, structural barriers, access to a telephone, and safety and hygiene practices.
• When assessing the patient's potential for complying with the treatment plan, consider such factors as history of psychiatric disorders, developmental status, substance abuse, comprehension, ability to read and write, and the presence of any language barriers.

Plan of care

Professional standards dictated by CHAP in 1993 — under the guidance of NLN — require you to develop a comprehensive plan of care in cooperation with the patient and his caregivers. In many aspects of care, the patient and family become the decision makers. This fact must be taken into account when developing your plan of care; adjust your interventions, patient goals, and teaching accordingly.

Don't go astray (without documenting it)

Legally speaking, a plan of care is the most direct evidence of your nursing judgment. If you outline a plan of care and then deviate from it, a court may decide that you strayed from a reasonable standard of care. So be sure to update your plan of care and make sure it fits the patient's needs.

Some agencies use the home health certification form and plan of care form (required for Medicare reimbursement) as the official plan of care for Medicare patients. Most home health agencies, however, require a separate plan of care. Some agencies use a multidisciplinary, integrated plan of care (see *Interdisciplinary care plan*, page 144).

Alternatively, individual plans may be used for each service provided to the patient. For example, individual plans may be developed for skilled nursing, physical therapy, occupational therapy, medical social worker, and home health aide services. Such plans can be tailored to meet the patient's needs and more accurately reflect the agency's method of operation.

Guidelines for use

To document most effectively on your plan of care, follow these suggestions:
• Keep a copy of the plan of care in the patient's home for easy reference by him and his family.
• Make sure the plan is comprehensive by including more than the patient's physiologic problems. Also chart about the home environment; the attitudes of the patient, family, and caregiver; and the resources needed.
• Document physical changes that need to be made in the patient's home for him to receive proper care. Help the family find the resources to implement them.
• Describe the primary caregiver, including whether or not he lives with the patient, their relationship, his age and physical ability, and his willingness to help the patient. The patient's well-being may depend on this person's abilities.
• Show in your documentation how you made the most of the patient's strengths and resources. Strengths include support systems, good health habits and coping behav-

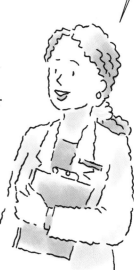

Don't forget to assess the patient's home environment and document your findings in the plan of care.

Art of the chart

Interdisciplinary care plan

The care plan is individualized for each patient. An example of this form is shown below.

Note that this care plan is focused on patient problems.

Set realistic goals.

Patient name: *Mary Long*

Primary nurse: *N. Smith, RN*

Init. cert. period: _____

Recert period #1: _____

Init. cert. period: _____

PROBLEM	GOAL	APPROACH	INITIAL CERT	RECERT #1	RECERT #2
Atrial fibrillation (10/1/97)	Maintain optimal cardiac output	1. Meds as ordered 2. Monitor vs, inc. apical rhythm and rate 3. observe for chest pain, dyspnea, palpitations, anxiety, etc.	GOAL MET? Y N INIT:_____	GOAL MET? Y N INIT:_____	GOAL MET? Y N INIT:_____
Heart Failure (12/1/97)	1. Maintain fluid and electrolyte balance 2. Promote optimal gas exchange.	1. Meds as ordered 2. Nebulizer as ordered 3. Draw labs as ordered 4. I & O daily 5. Monitor edema 6. ✔ for SOB, dyspnea, congestion (lung sounds) 7. amb. as tol 8. semi Fowler's when sitting	GOAL MET? Y N INIT:_____	GOAL MET? Y N INIT:_____	GOAL MET? Y N INIT:_____
Gastrostomy tube insertion (12/3/97)	1. Maintain optimal nutritional status 2. Prevent skin breakdown	1. Magnacal 80 ml/hr 2. Follow G-tube protocol, including site care & oral hygiene 3. Weekly weights 4. I&O daily 5. ✔ for N/V, diarrhea	GOAL MET? Y N INIT:_____	GOAL MET? Y N INIT:_____	GOAL MET? Y N INIT:_____

Intervention Codes
(please circle all that apply)

A1. Skilled observation
A2. Foley insertion
A3. Bladder installation
A4. Irrigation care (wd. dsg.)
A5. Irrigation decub. care - meds.
A6. Venipuncture
A7. Restorative nursing
A8. Postcataract care
A9. Bowel/Bladder training

A10. Chest physical (incl. postural drainage)
A11. Administer vit. B$_{12}$
A12. Prepare/Administer insulin
A13. Administer other
A14. Administer I.V.
A15. Teach ostomy care
A16. Teach nasogastric feeding
A17. Reposition nasogastric feeding tube
A18. Teach gastrostomy

A19. Teach parenteral nutrition
A20. Teach care of trach
A21. Administer care of trach
A22. Teach inhalation Rx
A23. Administer inhalation Rx
A24. Teach administration of injections
A25. Teach diabetic care
A26. Disimpaction/enema
A27. Other
   Foot care (diabetic)
   Teach diet
   Teach disease process

Teach use of 0$_2$
Instruct re: Medication child
A28. Wound care/dsg - closed
A29. Decubitus care - simple
A30. Teach care of indwelling catheter
A31. Management and evaluation of patient care plan
A32. Teaching and training (other)

Interventions are coded to allow for rapid documentation.

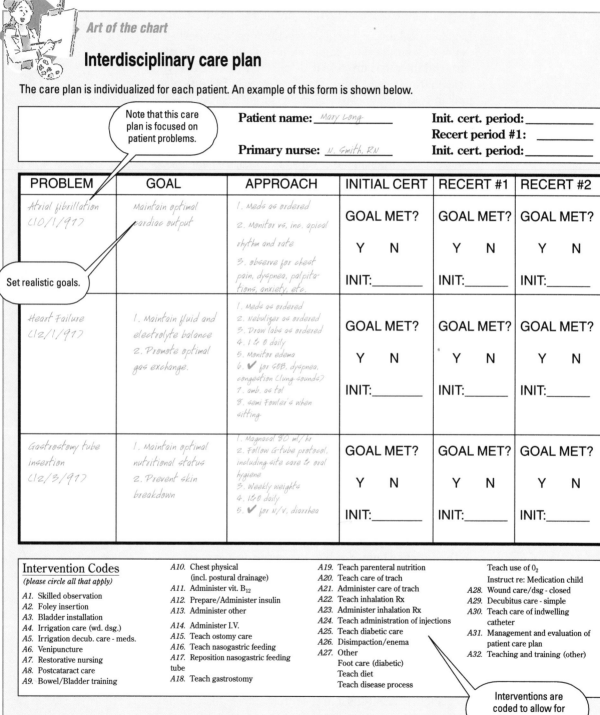

iors, a safe and healthful environment, and financial security. Resources include the doctor, pharmacy, and medical equipment supplier.

• If the patient is housebound, make sure this is documented and state the reason why. Medicare requires a patient receiving skilled home care to be housebound; however, some commercial insurers don't.

• Make sure that documentation reflects consistent adherence by all caregivers to the plan of care. Have caregivers demonstrate the procedures they use for the care they provide.

• Keep the record updated, noting changes in the patient's condition or plan of care, and document that you reported these changes to the doctor. Medicare, Medicaid, and certain other third-party payers won't reimburse for skilled services not reported to the doctor.

Progress notes

The home care progress note, like notes in the acute care setting, is a place to document both the patient's condition and significant events that occur while he is under your care. The progress note is written in chronological order based on each home visit. (See *Progress note*.)

Art of the chart

Progress note

Use this sample progress note as a guide when charting in home care settings.

Date	Problem no.	Problem title - subjective, objective, assessment, plan
11/14/91	#2	A: L foot stasis ulcer showing no improvement in size or amount of drainage since 11/1/91.
		P: Dr. Miller notified. Wound culture ordered and done. Will send specimen to lab. ———————— M. A. Ford, RN

Work in progress

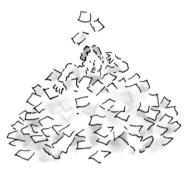

Every time you visit a patient, you must write a progress note. These notes document the following:
• changes in the patient's condition
• skilled nursing interventions you performed related to the plan of care
• the patient's responses to the interventions
• events or incidents in the home that might affect the treatment plan
• the patient's vital signs
• what you taught the patient and caregiver, including written instructional materials and brochures.

Guidelines for use

The guidelines below will help you chart safely and efficiently on progress notes:
• Chart all events in chronological order.
• Avoid addendums.
• Provide a heading for each entry because many members of the health care team use the progress notes.
• Use flow sheets and checklists to record vital signs, intake and output measurements, and nutritional data. Encourage the patient or caregiver to fill out these forms when appropriate. This gets them involved and increases their feeling of control.
• To help prevent the patient from feeling neglected, limit the time you spend charting in the home. When possible, take time to complete your charting while the patient sleeps or is otherwise occupied.
• Involve the patient in his own care and documentation by making statements like, "Here's what I've written about how your wound is healing. Is there anything else you want me to put in the notes?"
• If the patient has a medical emergency while you're there, accompany him to the hospital or emergency unit and stay until another caregiver takes over. Notify your supervisor, who will arrange coverage for your other patients, if necessary. Record all assessments and interventions performed until you're relieved. Note the date and time of transfer and the name of the caregiver who assumes responsibility.
• If documentation materials were completed and left in the patient's home, collect them at least once a week and

take them to your home health care agency. This keeps volumes of paper from piling up or becoming misplaced and also makes the records available for review by the agency supervisor.

Nursing and discharge summaries

As a home health nurse, you must submit a regular patient progress report to the attending doctor and the reimburser to confirm the need for continuing services. You must also complete a summary of the patient's progress and, when appropriate, a discharge summary.

Summing it all up

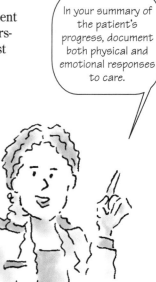

In your summary of the patient's progress, document both physical and emotional responses to care.

When writing a summary of the patient's progress, include the following information:
• current problems, treatments, interventions, and instructions
• home care provided by other health care professionals, such as a physical therapist or speech pathologist
• the reason for a change in services
• patient outcomes and responses — both physical and emotional — to the services provided.

Guidelines for use

You'll prepare a discharge summary to get the doctor's approval to discharge a patient, to notify third-party payers that services have been terminated, and to officially close the case. The discharge summary also serves as a brief history for quick review if the patient is readmitted at a later date. When writing these summaries, record:
• the time frame covered
• services provided and names and titles of assigned staff
• the third-party payer and whether or not the patient is eligible for future payment (he may have exhausted his annual benefits)
• the clinical and psychosocial condition of the patient at discharge
• recommendations for further care

• the patient's response to and comprehension of patient-teaching efforts
• outcomes attained.

Medicare-mandated forms

HCFA, the federal watchdog agency that oversees Medicare and Medicaid programs, requires home health agencies that receive Medicare funding to standardize their record-keeping and documentation methods. Home health agencies must maintain the following forms for each qualified Medicare recipient:
• home health certification and plan of care
• health update and patient information
• notice of nondiscrimination.

In addition, home care nurses must document a doctor's telephone orders. (See *Home health certification and plan of care; Medical update and patient information,* page 150; and *Doctor's telephone orders,* page 151.)

Fill out and sign, please . . .

Medicare won't pay unless the required forms are properly completed, signed, and submitted. Forms are usually filled out by the nurse assigned to the patient.

Future developments

Several major trends are emerging as the home health care industry continues to evolve.

More paperwork (surprise!)

More and more private insurers require preauthorization for home health care services, which increases the paperwork burden for nurses. Various payers may have different paperwork requirements and recertification periods, which can make managing the documenta-

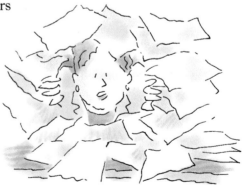

Art of the chart

Home health certification and plan of care

The form below is the official form for authorizing Medicare coverage for home care (also known as form 485). It includes space for assessing functional abilities and documenting plan of care information.

To maintain Medicare coverage, complete this form and submit for approval every 60 days.

Note that a patient is required to be housebound to receive Medicare reimbursement.

HOME HEALTH CERTIFICATION AND PLAN OF CARE

Form Approved
OMB No. 0938-0357

2. Start Of Care Date: 03/08/91	3. Certification Period From: 01/08/91 To: 09/08/91	4. Medical Record No. 78-9101	5. Provider No. 11-1213

1. Patient's HI Claim No. 111-111

6. Patient's Name and Address
Mary Long
2218 Central Ave.
Wichita, Kansas

7. Provider's Name, Address and Telephone Number
Home Health Agency
301 Main St.
Wichita, Kansas

9. Sex M ☐ F ☒

8. Date of Birth 06/04/29

11. ICD-9-CM Principal Diagnosis
42731 atrial fibrillation   Date 01/1/91

12. ICD-9-CM Surgical Procedure
0000 gastrostomy tube insertion   Date 03/2/91

13. ICD-9-CM Other Pertinent Diagnoses
4280 heart failure   03/1/91
496 chr airway obstruct   11/29/90

10. Medications: Dose/Frequency/Route (N)ew (C)hanged
digoxin 0.125 mg P.O. q.d.; Lasix 20 mg P.O. q.d.; Capoten 12.5 mg b.i.d.; Proventil warfarin 5 mg P.O. q.d.; inh 2 puffs q.i.d./p.r.n.; MVI one P.O. q.d.; FeSo₄ 325 mg q.d.; Ex St Tylenol 500 mg q4h p.r.n.; albuterol 0.5cc with 3cc ns via nebulizer b.i.d.; 325 mg aspirin 1 x daily

15. Safety Measures: prevent falls

14. DME and Supplies gastrostomy tube supplies, cane

16. Nutritional Req. magnacal 80 ml/hr

17. Allergies: NKA

18.B. Activities Permitted
1 ☐ Complete Bedrest
2 ☐ Bedrest BRP
3 ☒ Up As Tolerated
4 ☐ Transfer Bed/Chair
5 ☐ Exercises Prescribed
6 ☐ Partial Weight Bearing
7 ☐ Independent At Home
8 ☐ Crutches
9 ☒ Cane
A ☐ Wheelchair
B ☐ Walker
C ☐ No Restrictions
D ☐ Other (Specify)

18.A. Functional Limitations
1 ☐ Amputation
2 ☐ Bowel/Bladder (Incontinence)
3 ☐ Contracture
4 ☐ Hearing
5 ☐ Paralysis
6 ☒ Endurance
7 ☐ Ambulation
8 ☐ Speech
9 ☐ Legally Blind
A ☐ Dyspnea With Minimal Exertion
B ☐ Other (Specify)

19. Mental Status:
1 ☒ Oriented
2 ☐ Comatose
3 ☐ Forgetful
4 ☐ Depressed
5 ☐ Disoriented
6 ☐ Lethargic
7 ☐ Agitated
8 ☐ Other
3 ☐ Fair
4 ☒ Good
5 ☐ Excellent
1 ☐ Poor
2 ☐ Guarded

20. Prognosis:

21. Orders for Discipline and Treatments (Specify Amount/Frequency/Duration)
RN: assess heart failure, effects of digoxin, monitor complaints of arthritis pain control; monitor gastrostomy tube site, help with gastrostomy feedings and tube care. Draw blood as ordered by MD. AID 2-3 wk; assist with personal care and ADLs.

22. Goals/Rehabilitation Potential/Discharge Plans
Pt needs teaching, reinforcement and emotional support for colostomy. Rehab potential is good.
Skilled nursing facility.

23. Nurse's Signature and Date of Verbal SOC Where Applicable: N. Smith, RN 01/08/91

25. Date HHA Received Signed POT 01/08/91

24. Physician's Name and Address
M. Roser, MD
555 Main St.
Wichita, Kansas

26. I certify/recertify that this patient is confined to his/her home and needs intermittent skilled nursing care, physical therapy and/or speech therapy or continues to need occupational therapy. The patient is under my care, and I have authorized the services on this plan of care and will periodically review the plan.

27. Attending Physician's Signature and Date Signed
M. Roser, MD

28. Anyone who misrepresents, falsifies, or conceals essential information required for payment of Federal funds may be subject to fine, imprisonment, or civil penalty under applicable Federal laws.

PROVIDER

Form HCFA-485 (C-4) (02-94) (Print Aligned)

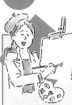

Art of the chart

Medical update and patient information

To continue providing reimbursable skilled nursing care to a patient at home, Medicare requires you to complete the Medical Update and Patient Information form (also known as form 486).

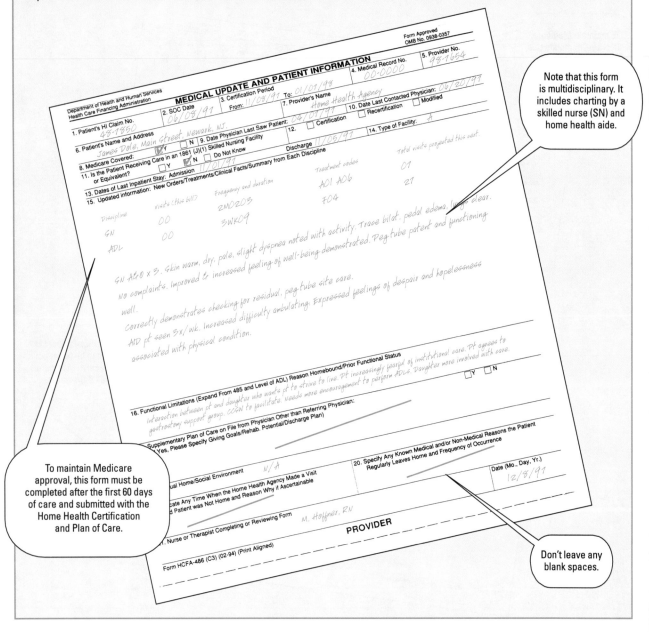

Note that this form is multidisciplinary. It includes charting by a skilled nurse (SN) and home health aide.

To maintain Medicare approval, this form must be completed after the first 60 days of care and submitted with the Home Health Certification and Plan of Care.

Don't leave any blank spaces.

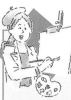

> *Art of the chart*

Doctor's telephone orders

Home health nurses rely heavily on the use of telephone orders. The agency must follow guidelines established by the Health Care Financing Administration for taking and documenting these orders. Below is an example of a form used by one agency to fulfill documentation requirements. The order must be signed by the doctor within 48 hours.

Facility name			Address		
Suburban Home Health Agency			*123 Main Street*		
Last name	**First name**		**Attending doctor**		**Admission no.**
Smith	*Kevin*		*Baker*		*147-111-471*

Date ordered	Date discontinued	ORDERS
12/18/91	*12/21/91*	*Tylenol 650 mg P.O. q6h p.r.n. Temp > 101° F*

Signature of nurse receiving order	Time	Signature of doctor	Date
Mary Reo, RN	*1820*		

tion requirements of a patient caseload confusing. In this cost-conscious environment, nurses may be confronted with ethical dilemmas about limitations on care imposed by cost considerations.

Bigger business

Over time, home health agencies will be forced to merge with hospital networks or coalitions of other home health agencies to form integrated delivery systems. The independent agency may cease to exist as insurance companies seek contracts only with agencies that can provide diverse services to a wide geographic area.

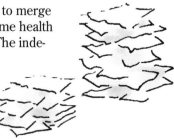

Outcomes are in

Increased reliance on disease-specific management programs will eventually lead to use of critical pathways that incorporate patient outcomes in home health care. In the future, the quality of an agency's services will be measured by disease-specific outcome data.

The keyboard approach

Increasingly, home health care nurses are using laptop computers equipped with software designed to speed clinical documentation. Many of these programs are designed to help nurses develop a plan of care, formulate goals, monitor patient progress, update medications, and generate visit notes. This technology expedites the exchange of data between care providers and third-party payers. Nurses inexperienced in using computers should be aware that documentation may take longer until they adjust to the new equipment.

Keeping it confidential

New technology raises new concerns about confidentiality. For example, e-mail and faxes can easily end up in the wrong hands. When using either to transmit information about a patient, consider blacking out identifying data. Arrange for the recipient of a fax to wait at the other end for the fax to print.

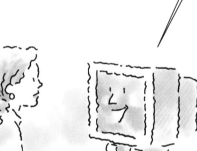

In many cases, a home health agency will supply its nurses with laptop computers to streamline documentation. Laptop computers shouldn't be used by anyone other than agency personnel. You may be tempted to allow a computer-savvy spouse, friend, or child to add programs or manipulate data with all good intentions, but this is no more appropriate than it would be to let them read a patient's record. Finally, access to computer files should be protected by password to prevent unauthorized individuals from entering files.

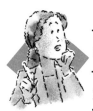

Quick quiz

1. The agency that requires standardized record keeping and documentation for Medicare recipients is:
- A. JCAHO.
- B. HCFA.
- C CHAP.

Answer: B. The Health Care Financing Administration requires that documentation and record keeping be standardized for Medicare reimbursement.

2. State nursing boards require home health agencies to annually update:
- A. policy and procedure manuals.
- B. nursing staff qualifications.
- C. desk calendars.

Answer: A. All state boards of nursing require that updated nursing policy and procedure manuals be available to staff.

3. Changes in the patient's condition should be documented:
- A. in the progress notes.
- B. in the plan of care.
- C. in the critical pathway.

Answer: A. Significant events that occur during your care of the patient are documented in the progress notes, which are maintained in chronological order based on each home visit.

4. The fact that a patient is housebound should be documented on the plan of care in order to:
- A. meet reimbursement requirements of commercial insurance companies.
- B. meet Medicare requirements for reimbursement.
- C. meet the reimbursement requirements of both Medicare and commercial insurance companies.

Answer: B. Medicare requires a patient receiving skilled home care to be housebound; however, some commercial insurers don't.

5. An important reason to encourage the patient and family members to fill out flow sheets and checklists is to:

      A. enable nurses and home health aides to provide care in less time.

      B. decrease the home health agency's liability risk.

      C. foster greater involvement in care.

Answer: C. Encouraging patient and family members to fill out these forms involves them in care activities and increases their feeling of control.

6. One drawback to transmitting patient information by e-mail or fax is that:

      A. it's hard to read.

      B. it threatens patient confidentiality.

      C. it causes duplication and redundancy.

Answer: B. Electronically transmitted data can easily fall into the wrong hands.

Scoring

☆☆☆ If you answered all six items correctly, turn off your laptop and hop into a hammock. Rest assured that you're home-free with documentation.

☆☆ If you answered four or five correctly, good for you! You meet all certification and utilization review requirements that will allow you to go on to the next chapter.

☆ If you answered fewer than four correctly, keep at it! You'll always come across new opportunities to use your charting know-how. Just turn to the next chapter and see.

7

Long-term care and rehabilitation

Just the facts

In this chapter, you'll learn:

♦ about agencies that regulate documentation in long-term care settings

♦ specific forms required in long-term care settings and how to complete them

♦ guidelines for correct documentation.

A look at charting in long-term care

A long-term care facility provides continuing care for chronically ill or disabled patients. The purpose of care is to promote the highest level of functioning possible for the patient. Long-term care is an increasingly important form of health care delivery, especially because the elderly segment of the population is rapidly growing. (See *Elder power,* page 156.)

Maintaining accurate, complete documentation in long-term care is vital. Consider the following points:

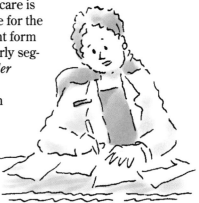

• Long-term care facilities are highly regulated by state and federal agencies and therefore must live up to high standards of documentation.

• Information in your records may be used to defend you and your facility in court.

• Your employer views documentation records as evidence of standardized, high-quality nursing care.

• Good record keeping ensures certification, licensure, reimbursement, and accreditation.

Elder power

Between 1960 and 1996, the U.S. population increased by 45% overall. However, the number of people age 65 and older grew by 100%, and the number of people age 85 and older increased by almost 300%. This last group — the "oldest old" — is the fastest-growing segment of our population. During the next 50 years, the number of people in this age group is expected to increase even more.

Chances are, you're caring for many elderly patients right now. Studies show that people age 65 and older require health care services more often than any other age group. In fact, they account for 30% of all hospital discharges and 36% of the country's personal health care expenditures. That's why we need to focus increasingly on the needs of the elderly in long-term nursing care (as well as in subacute and home care), and in inpatient and outpatient rehabilitative and psychiatric care.

There's strength in numbers!

Documentation distinctions

Two key differences exist between documenting in long-term care settings and other settings:

First, patients stay at long-term care facilities for weeks or months, so documentation isn't done as often. This takes the emphasis off charting and puts it on helping the patient relearn basic skills.

Second, some of the government forms used in long-term facilities are long and involved. So, even though charting isn't emphasized, it can still be extensive.

Categories of care

Long-term care facilities usually offer two levels of care: skilled and intermediate. The level of care administered to your patient should be your primary consideration when documenting.

Care may be complex...

In a skilled care facility, patient care involves specialized nursing skills, such as I.V. therapy, parenteral nutrition, respiratory care, and mechanical ventilation.

...or not so complex

An intermediate care facility deals with patients who have chronic illnesses and need less complex care. For exam-

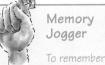

ple, they may simply need assistance with activities of daily living (ADLs), such as bathing and dressing.

Patients at both levels may need short- or long-term care and may move from one level to another according to their progress or decline. Living arrangements, geography, family and community support networks, and other factors determine the patient's length of stay.

Regulatory agencies

Documentation in long-term care facilities is regulated by both federal and state agencies. Documentation is influenced by:
• federal programs, such as Medicare and Medicaid
• government agencies such as the Health Care Financing Administration (HCFA)
• laws such as the Omnibus Budget Reconciliation Act (OBRA) of 1987.
• state regulations for each facility.

Most elderly patients entering a long-term care facility pay for the services privately. When their funds become exhausted, they apply to Medicaid for coverage. If the patient requires services and is unable to pay initially, he can apply to receive Medicaid.

> **Memory Jogger**
>
> To remember the conditions that affect length of stay, think of the word FOCUS:
>
> • Functional skills (and disabilities)
> • Other diseases
> • Chronicity
> • Urgency of needs
> • Support systems.

Medicare

Few of the services provided in long-term care facilities are eligible for Medicare reimbursement. However, Medicare does provide reimbursement for patients requiring skilled care, such as chemotherapy or tube feeding. For these patients, Medicare requires certain minimum daily documentation to prove that a service was needed. If the patient's status changes, you must supply a revised plan of care within 7 days.

Making reimbursement a reality

Be sure to document changes in status, because when a patient isn't improving or isn't expected to improve according to his plan of care, he becomes ineligible for coverage. You must also document the need for any new or continuing skilled services you provide. Medicare also re-

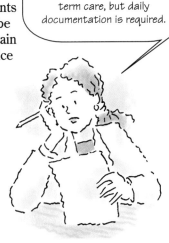

Medicare does cover some skilled services in long-term care, but daily documentation is required.

quires documentation of your evaluations for expected outcomes.

According to Medicare guidelines, charting must clearly show that a patient needed care by a professional or technical staff member. To verify the need for skilled rehabilitative care, you must describe a reasonable expectation of improvement or services needed to establish a maintenance program. The amount, duration, and frequency of services must be reasonable and necessary.

Medicaid

Most patients who receive skilled care in long-term care facilities either pay for it themselves or are on Medicaid. To ensure Medicaid reimbursement for these patients, document patient care once a day.

Reimbursement for intermediate care

To secure payment for patients receiving intermediate care, medications and treatments are documented daily. Document other types of care weekly unless the patient's status changes and he requires a change in services. In this case, chart the change and document his status more frequently. Also perform a monthly reevaluation for these patients and an evaluation of expected outcomes for all Medicaid patients.

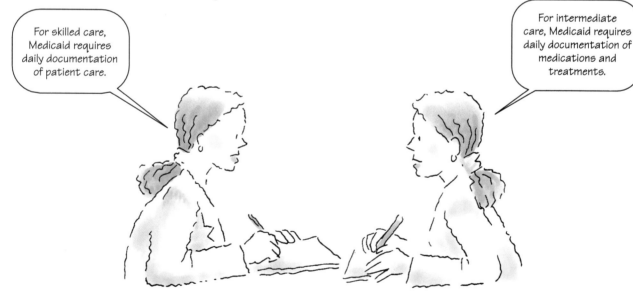

For skilled care, Medicaid requires daily documentation of patient care.

For intermediate care, Medicaid requires daily documentation of medications and treatments.

HCFA

A branch of the Department of Health and Human Services, HCFA regulates compliance with federal Medicare and Medicaid standards. HCFA regulations are usually enforced at the state level.

To comply with HCFA regulations, staff members at a long-term care facility must complete a lengthy form called the Minimum Data Set for Resident Assessment and Care Screening (MDS), review the patient's status every 3 months, and perform a comprehensive reassessment annually.

OBRA

In 1987, Congress enacted the Omnibus Budget Reconciliation Act, which imposed dozens of new requirements on long-term care facilities and home health agencies to protect the rights of patients receiving long-term care. OBRA requires that a comprehensive assessment be performed within 4 days of a patient's admission to a long-term care facility and then be charted on the MDS form. The assessment and care screening process must be reviewed every 3 months and repeated annually; more often if the patient's condition changes.

In addition, a comprehensive nursing assessment and a formulated plan of care must be completed within 7 days of admission.

Forms used in long-term care

Many forms are used in both acute care and home health care settings as well as in long-term care; others are used only in long-term care. Forms discussed in this chapter include:
• MDS
• Resident Assessment Protocol (RAP)
• Preadmission Screening and Annual Resident Review (PASARR)
• initial nursing assessment form
• nursing summaries

• ADL checklists or flow sheets
• plans of care
• discharge and transfer forms.

In addition, many long-term care facilities have their own strict and comprehensive protocols. Typical protocols are those for bowel and bladder monitoring, physical and chemical restraints, safety, and infection control. Charting requirements when using these protocols vary, so check your facility's policies.

Minimum Data Set

Mandated by OBRA, this federal regulatory form must be filled out for every patient admitted to a long-term care facility. (See *Minimum Data Set form.*)

The MDS form proves compliance with quality improvement and reimbursement requirements, standardizes information, and helps health care team members and agencies communicate. Doctors, nurses, social workers, and other staff members complete and sign different sections of the form.

Resident Assessment Protocol

Once an MDS form is completed, coded, computed, and processed, the patient's primary problems can be identified. These problems provide the basis for the patient's plan of care. Another federally mandated form, the RAP summary lists identified problem areas and documents the existence of a corresponding plan of care. For example, if the patient has a stage 2 pressure ulcer documented in the MDS, the RAP summary indicates the need for a plan of care to treat the pressure ulcer. (See *Resident Assessment Protocol Summary*, page 166.)

The RAP summary documents patient problems and the existence of a plan of care.

PASARR

A patient's mental status must also be documented to qualify for Medicare or Medicaid reimbursement. Federal regulations require long-term care facilities to perform a complete mental status assessment and document it on a

(Text continues on page 167.)

Art of the chart

Minimum Data Set form

Patients in long-term care facilities that receive federal funds must have their health status evaluated at admission and a plan of care devised. The patient's health status and plan of care are revised every 7 days. The following form is used for reevaluation.

SECTION A. IDENTIFICATION AND BACKGROUND INFORMATION

1. ASSESSMENT DATE	[1 1] [0 1] [1 9 9 1] Month Day Year
2. RESIDENT NAME	*Cary* *L.* *Gallen* (First) (Middle Initial) (Last)
3. SOCIAL SECURITY #	[1 9 4] — [5 0] — [3 5 2 2]
(MEDICAID) (if applicable)	[ ]
	[M M 0 0 0 9 9 2 2 6 5 1]
...FOR ...ESSMENT	1. Initial admission assess 5. Significant 2. Hosp/Medicare reassess change in status 3. Readmission assess 6. Other (e.g., UR) 4. Annual assess [ ]
7. CURRENT PAYMENT SOURCE(S) FOR N.H. STAY	*(Billing office to indicate: check all that apply)* Medicaid [A.] VA [D.] Medicare [B.✔] Self pay/Private insurance [E.✔] CHAMPUS [C.] Other [F.]
8. RESPON-SIBILITY/LEGAL GUARDIAN	*(Check all that apply)* Legal guardian [A.✔] Family member responsible [D.✔] Other legal oversight [B.] Resident responsible [E.] Durable power attrny/health care proxy [C.] NONE OF ABOVE [F.]
9. ADVANCE DIRECTIVES	*(For those items with supporting documentation in the medical record, check all that apply)* Living will [A.✔] Feeding restrictions [F.] Do not resuscitate [B.✔] Medication restrictions [G.] Do not hospitalize [C.] Other treatment Organ donation [D.] restrictions [H.✔] Autopsy request [E.] NONE OF ABOVE [I.]
10. DISCHARGE PLANNED WITHIN 3 MOS.	(Does not include discharge due to death) 0. No 1. Yes 2. Unknown/Uncertain [ ]
11. PARTICIPATE IN ASSESSMENT	A. Resident B. Family [A.] 0. No 1. Yes 0. No 1. Yes 2. No family [B.]
12. SIGNATURES	Signature of RN Assessment Coordinator *Sarah Rios, RN* Signatures of others who completed *Renee Meeh RN* *Edward Solis MSW* *Eileen Clantz MD*

Place resident's name and the date on each assessment.

Assess mental status.

[gray box] = Code the appropriate response   [ ] = Check all responses that apply

SECTION B. COGNITIVE PATTERNS

1. COMATOSE	0. No 1. Yes *(Skip to SECTION E)* [0]
2. MEMORY	*(Recall of what was learned or known)* A. Short-term memory OK–seems/appears to recall after 5 minutes 0. Memory OK 1. Memory problem [A. 1] B Long-term memory OK–seems/appears to recall long past 0. Memory OK 1. Memory problem [B. 1]
3. MEMORY/ RECALL ABILITY	*(Check all that resident normally able to recall during last 7 days)* Current season [A.] That he/she is in Location of own room [B.] a nursing home [D.✔] Staff names/faces NONE OF ABOVE [E.] are recalled [C.]
4. COGNITIVE SKILLS FOR DAILY DECISION-MAKING	*(Made decisions regarding tasks of daily life)* 0. Independent–decisions consistent/reasonable 1. Modified independence–some difficulty in new situations only 2. Moderately impaired–decisions poor; cues/supervision required 3. Severely impaired–never/rarely made decisions [3]
5. INDICATIONS OF DELIRIUM– PERIODIC DISORDERED THINKING/ AWARENESS	*(Check if condition over last 7 days different from usual functioning)* Less alert, easily distracted [A.] Changing awareness of environment [B.] Episodes of incoherent speech [C.] Periods of motor restlessness or lethargy [D.] Cognitive ability varies over course of day [E.] NONE OF ABOVE [F.✔]
6. CHANGE IN COGNITIVE STATUS	Change in resident's cognitive status, skills, or abilities in last 90 days 0. No 1. Improved 2. Deteriorated [0]

SECTION C. COMMUNICATION/HEARING PATTERNS

1. HEARING	*(With hearing appliance, if used)* 0. Hears adequately–normal talk, TV, phone 1. Minimal difficulty when not in quiet setting 2. Hears in special situations only–speaker has to adjust tonal quality and speak distinctly 3. Highly impaired/absence of useful hearing [2]
2. COMMUNI-CATION DEVICES/ TECHNIQUES	*(Check all that apply during last 7 days)* Hearing aid present and used [A.] Hearing aid present and not used [B.✔] Other receive comm. techniques used (e.g., lip read) [C.] NONE OF ABOVE [D.]

Use check marks to identify relevant information.

(continued)

Minimum Data Set form *(continued)*

3. MODES OF EXPRESSION	*(Check all used by resident to make needs known)*
	Speech A. ✔ Signs/gestures/sounds C. ☐ Writing messages Communication board D. ☐ to express or Other E. ☐ clarify needs B. ☐ *NONE OF ABOVE* F. ☐

4. MAKING SELF UNDERSTOOD	*(Express information content–however able)* 0. Understood 1. Usually understood–difficulty finding words, finishing thoughts 2. Sometimes understood–ability is limited to making concrete requests 3. Rarely/Never understood

5. ABILITY TO UNDERSTAND OTHERS	*(Understanding verbal information content–however able)* 0. Understands 1. Usually understands–may miss some part/intent of message 2. Sometimes understands–responds adequately to simple, direct communication 3. Rarely/Never understands ☐ 2

6. CHANGE IN COMMUNI-CATION/ HEARING	Resident's ability to express, understand or hear information has changed *over last 90 days* 0. No change 1. Improved 2. Deteriorated ☐ 0

SECTION D. VISION PATTERNS

1. VISION	*(Ability to see in adequate light and glasses if used)* 0. Adequate–sees fine detail, including regular print in newspapers/books 1. Impaired–sees large print, but not regular print in newspapers/books 2. Highly impaired–limited vision; not able to see newspaper headlines; appears to follow objects with eyes 3. Severely impaired–no vision or appears to see only light, colors, or shapes ☐ 2

2. VISION LIMITATIONS/ DIFFICULTIES	A. Side vision problems–decreased peripheral vision (e.g., leaves food on one side of tray, difficulty traveling, bumps into people and objects, misjudges placement of chair when seating self) B. Experiences any of the following: sees halos or rings around lights; sees flashes of light; sees "curtains" over eyes C. *NONE OF ABOVE* ☐ C

3. VISUAL APPLIANCES	Glasses; contact lenses; lens implant; magnifying glass 0. No 1. Yes ☐ 1

SECTION E. PHYSICAL FUNCTIONING AND STRUCTURAL PROBLEMS

1. ADL SELF-PERFORMANCE–*(Code for resident's PERFORMANCE OVER ALL SHIFTS during last 7 days–Not including setup)*   0. *INDEPENDENT*–no help or oversight–OR–Help/Oversight provided only 1 or 2 times during last 7 days   1. *SUPERVISION*–Oversight, encouragement or cueing provided 3+ times during last 7 days   2. *LIMITED ASSISTANCE*–Resident highly involved in activity; received physical help in guided maneuvering of limbs or other nonweight bearing assistance 3+ times–OR–More help provided only 1 or 2 times during last 7 days   3. *EXTENSIVE ASSISTANCE*–While resident performed part of activity, over last 7-day period, help of the following type(s) provided 3 or more times: –Weight-bearing support   –Full staff performance during part (but not all) of last 7 days   4. *TOTAL DEPENDENCE*–Full staff performance of activity during entire 7 days

This section covers activities of daily living.

This scale is for rating functional ability.

2. ADL SUPPORT PROVIDED–*(Code for MOST SUPPORT PROVIDED OVER ALL SHIFTS during last 7 days; code regardless of resident's self-performance classification)* 0. No setup or physical help from staff 1. Setup help only 2. One-person physical assist 3. Two-person physical assist		(1) SELF-PERF.	(2) SUPPORT
A. BED MOBILITY	How resident moves to and from lying position, turns side to side, and positions body while in bed	3	3
B. TRANSFER	How resident moves between surfaces–to/from: bed, chair, wheelchair, standing position (EXCLUDE to/from bath/toilet)	4	3
C. LOCO-MOTION	How resident moves between locations in his/her room and adjacent corridor on same floor; if in wheelchair, self-sufficiency once in chair	3	2
D. DRESSING	How resident puts on, fastens, and takes off all items of street clothing, including donning/removing prosthesis	4	3
E. EATING	How resident eats and drinks (regardless of skill)	2	2
F. TOILET USE	How resident uses the toilet room (or commode, bedpan, urinal); transfer on/off toilet, cleanses, changes pad, manages ostomy or catheter, adjusts clothes	4	3
G. PERSONAL HYGIENE	How resident maintains personal hygiene, including combing hair, brushing teeth, shaving, applying makeup, washing/drying face, hands, and perineum (EXCLUDE baths and showers)	3	2
3. BATHING	How resident takes full-body bath/shower, sponge bath and transfers in/out of tub/shower (EXCLUDE washing of back and hair. **Code for most dependent** in self-performance and support. Bathing Self-Performance codes appear below.) 0. Independent–No help provided 1. Supervision–Oversight help only 2. Physical help limited to transfer only 3. Physical help in part of bathing activity 4. Total dependence A. 3 B. 3		

4. BODY CONTROL PROBLEMS	*(Check all that apply during last 7 days)*
	Balance–partial or total loss of ability to balance self while standing A. ✔ Bedfast all or most of the time B. ☐ Contracture to arms, legs, shoulders, or hands C. ☐ Quadriplegia D. ☐ Arm–partial or total loss of voluntary movement E. ✔ Hand–lack of dexterity (e.g. problem using tooth brush or adjusting hearing aid) F. ✔ Leg–partial or total loss of voluntary movement G. ✔ Leg–unsteady gait H. ☐ Trunk–partial or total loss of ability to position, balance, or turn body I. ✔ Amputation J. ✔ *NONE OF ABOVE* K. ☐

5. TASK SEG-MENTATION	Resident requires that some or all of ADL activities be broken into a series of subtasks so that resident can perform them 0. No 1. Yes ☐ 1

Minimum Data Set form (continued)

6. MOBILITY APPLIANCES/ DEVICES	(Check all that apply during last 7 days)		
	Cane walker	A.	Other person wheeled	D. ✔
	Brace/prosthesis	B.	Lifted (manually/	
	Wheeled self	C.	mechanically)	E. ✔
			NONE OF ABOVE	

7. ADL FUNCTIONAL REHABILITATION POTENTIAL	Resident believes he/she capable of increased independence in at least some ADLs	
	Direct care staff believe resident capable of increased independence in at least some ADL	
	Resident able to perform tasks/activity but is very slow	
	Major difference in ADL Self-Performance or ADL Support in mornings and evenings (at least a one category change in Self-Performance or Support in any ADL)	D.
	NONE OF ABOVE	E.

8. CHANGE IN ADL FUNCTION	Change in ADL self-performance in last 90 days	
	0. No change 1. Improved 2. Deteriorated	0

SECTION F. CONTINENCE IN LAST 14 DAYS

1. CONTINENCE SELF-CONTROL CATEGORIES
(Code for resident performance over all shifts)
0. CONTINENT–Complete control
1. USUALLY CONTINENT–BLADDER, incontinent episodes once a week or less; BOWEL, less than weekly
2. OCCASIONALLY INCONTINENT–BLADDER, 2+ times a week but not daily; BOWEL, once a week
3. FREQUENTLY INCONTINENT– BLADDER, tended to be incontinent daily, but some control present (e.g. on day shift); BOWEL, 2-3 times a week
4. INCONTINENT– Had inadequate control, BLADDER, multiple daily episodes; BOWEL, all (or almost all) of the time

A. BOWEL CONTINENCE	Control of bowel movement, with appliance or bowel continence programs, if employed	4
B. BLADDER CONTINENCE	Control of urinary bladder function (if dribbles, volume insufficient to soak through underpants), with appliances (e.g., foley) or continence programs if employed	4

2. INCONTINENCE RELATED TESTING	(Skip if resident's bladder continence code equals 0 or 1 AND no catheter is used)	
	Resident has been tested for a urinary tract infection	A. ✔
	Resident has been checked for presence of a fecal impaction, or there is adequate bowel elimination	B. ✔
	NONE OF ABOVE	C.

3. APPLIANCES PROGRAMS	Any scheduled toileting plan	A.	Pads/Briefs used	F.
	External (condom) catheter	B.	Enemas/Irrigation	G.
	Indwelling catheter	C. ✔	Ostomy	H.
	Intermittent catheter	D.	NONE OF ABOVE	I.
	Did not use toilet room/ commode/urinal	E.		

4. CHANGE IN URINARY CONTINENCE	Change in urinary continence/appliances and programs **in last 90 days**	
	0. No change 1. Improved 2. Deteriorated	2

SECTION G. PSYCHOSOCIAL WELL-BEING

1. SENSE OF INITIATIVE/ INVOLVEMENT	At ease interacting with others	A. ✔
	At ease doing planned or structural activities	B.
	At ease doing self-initiated activities	C.
	Establishes own goals	D.
	Pursues involvement in life of facility (e.g. makes/ keeps friends; involved in group activities; responds positively to new activities; assists at religious services)	E.
	Accepts invitations into most group activities	F. ✔
	NONE OF ABOVE	G.

This section covers psychosocial status.

2. UNSETTLED RELATIONSHIPS	Covert/Open conflict with and/or repeated criticism of staff	A.
	Unhappy with roommate	B.
	Unhappy with residents other than roommate	C.
	Openly expresses conflict/anger with family or friends	D.
	Absence of personal contact with family/friends	E. ✔
	Recent loss of close family member/friend	F. ✔
	NONE OF ABOVE	G.

3. PAST ROLES	Strong identification with past roles and life status	A.
	Expresses sadness/anger/empty feeling over lost roles/status	B. ✔
	NONE OF ABOVE	C.

SECTION H. MOOD AND BEHAVIOR PATTERNS

1. SAD OR ANXIOUS MOOD	(Check all that apply during last 30 days)	
	VERBAL EXPRESSIONS of DISTRESS by resident (sadness, sense that nothing matters, hopelessness, worthlessness, unrealistic fears, vocal expressions of anxiety or grief)	A.
	DEMONSTRATED (OBSERVABLE) SIGNS of mental DISTRESS	
	–Tearfullness, emotional groaning, sighing, breathlessness	B. ✔
	–Motor agitation, such as pacing, handwringing or picking	C.
	–Failure to eat or take medications, withdrawal from self-care or leisure activities	D.
	–Pervasive concern about health	E.
	–Recurrent thoughts of death–e.g. believes he/she about to die, have a heart attack	F.
	–Suicidal thoughts/actions	G.
	NONE OF ABOVE	H.

2. MOOD PERSISTENCE	Sad or anxious mood intrudes on daily life over last 7 days–not easily altered, doesn't "cheer up"	
	0. No 1. Yes	0

3. RESIDENT RESISTS CARE	(Check all types of resistance that occurred in the last 7 days)	
	Resisted taking medications/injection	A.
	Resisted ADL assistance	B.
	NONE OF ABOVE	C. ✔

4. CHANGE IN MOOD	Change in mood **in last 90 days**	
	0. No change 1. Improved 2. Deteriorated	0

(continued)

This form is long but check marks and codes will help you save time.

Minimum Data Set form *(continued)*

5. PROBLEM BEHAVIOR	*(Code for behavior* in last 7 days)
	0. Behavior not exhibited in last 7 days 1. Behavior of this type occurred less than daily 2. Behavior of this type occurred daily or more frequently WANDERING (moved with no rational purpose, seemingly oblivious to needs or safety) — A. ⊘ VERBALLY ABUSIVE (others were threatened, screamed at, cursed at) — B. ⊘ PHYSICALLY ABUSIVE (others were hit, shoved, scratched, sexually abused) — C. ⊘ SOCIALLY INAPPROPRIATE/DISRUPTIVE BEHAVIOR (made disrupting sounds, noisy, screams, self-abusive acts, sexual behavior, disrobing in public, smeared/threw food/feces, hoarding, rummaging through others belongings) — D. ⊘

This section identifies problem behaviors.

6. BEHAVIOR MANAGEMENT PROGRAM	Behavior problem has been addressed by clinically developed behavior management program. (Note: Do not include programs that involve only physical restraint or psychotropic medications in this category) 0. No behavior problem 1. Yes, addressed 2. No, not addressed
7. CHANGE IN BEHAVIOR PROBLEM	Change in mood **in last 90 days** 0. No change 1. Improved 2. Deteriorated ⊘

SECTION I. ACTIVITY PURSUIT PATTERNS

1. TIME AWAKE	*(Check appropriate time periods* over last 7 days) Resident awake all or most of time (i.e., naps no more than one hour per time period) in the: Morning — A. ✔ Evening — C. ✔ Afternoon — B. *NONE OF ABOVE* — D.
2. AVERAGE TIME IN-VOLVED IN ACTIVITIES	0. Most—more than ⅔ of time 2. Little—less than ⅓ of time 1. Some—⅓ to ⅔ of time 3. None ▢
3. PREFERRED ACTIVITY SETTINGS	*(Check all settings* in which activities are preferred) Own room — A. Outside facility — C. Day/activity room — B. *NONE OF ABOVE* Inside NH/off unit — C.
4. GENERAL ACTIVITY PREFER-ENCES (adapted to resident's current abilities)	*(Check all PREFERENCES* whether or not activity is currently available to resident) Cards/Other games — A. Religious activities — F. ✔ Crafts/Arts — B. ✔ Trips/Shopping — G. ✔ Exercise/Sports — C. Walking/Wheeling outdoors — H. ✔ Music — D. ✔ Watch TV — I. ✔ Read/Write — E. *NONE OF ABOVE* — J.
5. PREFERS MORE OR DIFFERENT ACTIVITIES	Resident expresses/indicates preferences for other activities/choices 0. No 1. Yes ▢

SECTION J. DISEASE DIAGNOSES

Check only those diseases present that have a relationship to current ADL status, cognitive status, behavior status, medical treatments, or risk of death. (Do not list old/inactive diagnoses.)

1. DISEASES	*(If none apply, CHECK the NONE OF ABOVE box)*

	HEART/CIRCULATION **PSYCHIATRIC /MOOD**
	Arteriosclerotic heart disease (ASHD) — A. ✔ Anxiety disorder — P.
	Cardiac dysrhythmias — B. Depression — Q. ✔
	Congestive heart failure — C. Manic depressive (bipolar disease) — R.
	Hypertension — D. ✔ **SENSORY**
	Hypotension — E. Cataracts — S.
	Peripheral vascular disease — F. ✔ Glaucoma — T.
	Other cardiovascular disease — G. **OTHER**
	NEUROLOGIC Allergies — U.
	Alzheimer's — H. Anemia — V.
	Dementia other than Alzheimer's — I. Arthritis — W. ✔
	Aphasia — J. Cancer — X.
	Cerebrovascular accident (stroke) — K. Diabetes mellitus — Y.
	Multiple sclerosis — L. Explicit terminal prognosis — Z.
	Parkinson's disease — M. Hypothyroidism — AA. ✔
	PULMONARY Osteoporosis — BB.
	Emphysema/Asthma/ COPD — N. Seizure disorder — CC.
	Pneumonia — O. Septicemia — DD.
	   Urinary tract infection– (in last 30 days) — EE.
	   NONE OF ABOVE — FF.

2. OTHER CURRENT DIAGNOSES AND ICD-9 CODES	A. _Renal failure_ ▢▢▢ B. ___ C. ___ D. ___ E. ___ F. ___

List other diseases here.

SECTION K. HEALTH PROBLEMS

1. PROBLEM CONDITIONS	*(Check all problems* that are present in last 7 days unless other time frame indicated) Constipation — A. ✔ Pain–resident complains or shows evidence of pain daily or almost daily — J. Diarrhea — B. Dizziness/vertigo — C. Edema — D. Fecal impaction — E. Recurrent lung aspirations in last 90 days — K. Fever — F. Hallucinations/ Delusions — G. Shortness of breath — L. Syncope (fainting) — M. Internal bleeding — H. Vomiting — N. Joint pain — I. *NONE OF ABOVE* — O.
2. ACCIDENTS	Fell in past 30 days — A. Hip fracture in last 180 days — C. Fell in past 31-180 days — B.
3. STABILITY OF CONDITIONS	Conditions/Diseases make resident's cognitive, ADL, or behavior status unstable–fluctuating, precarious, or deteriorating — A. Resident experiencing an acute episode or a flare-up of a recurrent/chronic problem — B. ✔ *NONE OF ABOVE* — C.

Identify other health problems here.

Minimum Data Set form *(continued)*

1. ORAL PROBLEMS		
	Chewing problem	A.
	Swallowing problem	B.
	Mouth pain	C.
	NONE OF ABOVE	D. ✓

2. HEIGHT AND WEIGHT	
	Record height (A.) in inches and weight (B.) in pounds. Weight based on most recent status in last 30 days, measure weight consistently in accord with standard facility practice—e.g. in a.m., after voiding, before meal, with shoes off, and in nightclothes.
	HT. (in.) a. 6 4 WT. (lb.) b. 1 7 0
	(C.) Weight loss (i.e. 5%+ in **last 30 days**; or 10% in **last 180 days**) 0. No 1. Yes c.

3. NUTRITIONAL PROBLEMS		
	Complains about the taste of many foods	A. ✓
	Insufficient fluid; dehydrated	B.
	Did NOT consume all/almost all liquids provided during last 3 days	C.
	Regular complaint of hunger	D.
	Leaves 25%+ food uneaten at most meals	E. ✓
	NONE OF ABOVE	F.

4. NUTRITIONAL APPROACHES			
	Parenteral/I.V. A.	Therapeutic diet	E. ✓
	Feeding tube B.	Dietary supplement between meals	F.
	Mechanically altered diet C.	Plate guard, stabilized built-up utensil, etc.	G.
	Syringe (oral feeding tube) D.	*NONE OF ABOVE*	H.

SECTION M. ORAL/DENTAL STATUS

1. ORAL STATUS AND DISEASE PREVENTION		
	Debris (soft, easily movable substances) present in mouth prior to going to bed at night	A.
	Has dentures and/or removable bridge	B. ✓
	Some/all natural teeth lost–does not have or does not use dentures (or partial plates)	C.
	Broken, loose, or carious teeth	D.
	Inflamed gums (gingiva); swollen or bleeding gums; oral abscesses; ulcers or rashes	E.
	Daily cleaning of teeth/dentures	F. ✓
	NONE OF ABOVE	G.

> A detailed scale helps you assess pressure ulcers.

SECTION N. SKIN CONDITION

1. STASIS ULCER	
	(Open lesion caused by poor circulation to lower extremities) 0. No 1. Yes

2. PRESSURE ULCERS	
	(Code for highest stage of pressure ulcer)
	0. No pressure ulcers
	1. Stage 1-A persistent area of skin redness (without a break in skin) that does not disappear when pressure is relieved
	2. Stage 2-A partial thickness loss of skin layers that presents clinically as an abrasion, blister, or shallow crater
	3. Stage 3-A full thickness of skin lost, exposing the subcutaneous tissues–presents as a deep crater with or without undermining adjacent tissue
	4. Stage 4-A full thickness of skin and subcutaneous tissue lost, exposing muscle and/or bone 0

3. HISTORY OF RESOLVED/ CURED PRESSURE ULCERS	
	Resident has had pressure ulcer that was resolved/cured **in last 90 days** 0. No 1. Yes

4. SKIN PROBLEMS/ CARE		
	Open lesions other than stasis or pressure ulcers (e.g., cuts)	A.
	Skin desensitized to pain, pressure, discomfort	B.
	Protective/preventive skin care	C. ✓
	Turning/repositioning program	D. ✓
	Pressure relieving beds, bed/chair pads, (e.g., egg crate pads)	E.
	Wound care/treatment (e.g., pressure ulcer care, surgical wound)	F. ✓
	Other skin care/treatment	G. ✓
	NONE OF ABOVE	H.

SECTION O. MEDICATION USE

1. NUMBER OF MEDICATIONS	
	(Record the number of different medications used in the last 7 days; enter "0" if none used) 1 0

2. NEW MEDICATIONS	
	Resident has received new medications during the last 90 days 0. No 1. Yes 1

3. INJECTIONS	
	(Record the number of days injections of any type received during last 7 days) 2

4. DAYS RECEIVED THE FOLLOWING MEDICATION		
	(Record the number of days during the last 7 days; enter "0" if not used; enter "1" if long-acting meds. used less than weekly)	
	Antipsychotics	A. 0
	Antianxiety/Hypnotics	B. 0
	Antidepressants	C. 2

5. PREVIOUS MEDICATION RESULTS	
	(Skip this question if resident currently receiving antipsychotics, antidepressants, or antianxiety/hypnotics–otherwise code correct response for last 90 days)
	Resident has previously received psychoactive medications for a mood or behavior problem, and these medications were effective (without undue adverse consequences)
	0. No, drugs not used 2. Drugs were not effective 1. Drugs were effective 3. Drug effectiveness unknown

SECTION P. SPECIAL TREATMENT AND PROCEDURES

1. SPECIAL TREATMENTS AND PROCEDURES				
	SPECIAL CARE–*Check treatments received during last 14 days*			
	Chemotherapy	A.	I.V. meds	F. ✓
	Radiation	B.	Transfusions	G.
	Dialysis	C.	O2	H.
	Suctioning	D.	Other _____	I.
	Trach. care	E.	*NONE OF ABOVE*	J.
	THERAPIES–*Record the number of days* each of the following therapies was administered (for at least 10 minutes during a day) in the last 7 days:			
	Speech–language pathology and audiology services			K. 0
	Occupational therapy			L. 4
	Physical therapy			M. 3
	Psychological therapy			N.
	Respiratory therapy			O.

2. DEVICES AND RESTRAINTS				
	Use the following codes for last 7 days:			
	0. Not used 1. Used less than daily 2. Used daily			
	Bed rails	A. 2	Limb restraint	C. 0
	Trunk restraint	B. 0	Chair prevents rising	D. 0

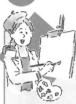

Art of the chart

Resident Assessment Protocol Summary

After recording the certification data on the MDS form, analyze it to identify the patient's primary problems and care needs. Then fill in the Resident Assessment Protocol (RAP) Summary shown below. The completed form verifies that you've written a plan of care.

Resident's name: *Leo Mancuso*   Medical record no.: *0839-2541*

Signature of RN assessment coordinator: *M. Burns, RN, BSN*

> Your signature here

RESIDENT ASSESSMENT PROTOCOL SUMMARY

1. For each RAP area triggered, show whether you are proceeding with a care plan intervention.

2. Document problems, complications, and risk factors; the need for referral to appropriate health care professionals: and the reasons for deciding to proceed or not to proceed to care planning. Documentation may appear anywhere the facility routinely keeps such information, such as problem sheets or progress notes.

3. Identify the location of this information.

RAP problem area	Care planning decision		Location of information
	Proceed	Do not proceed	
Delirium	☐	☑	*N/A See neuro note 11/2/91*
Cognitive loss and dementia	☑	☐	*Plan of Care #1*
Visual function	☑	☐	*Plan of Care #3*
Communication	☑	☐	*Plan of Care #3*
ADL functional and rehabilitation potential	☑	☐	*Plan of Care #3*
Urinary incontinence and indwelling catheter	☑	☐	*Plan of Care #4*
Psychosocial well-being	☑	☐	*Plan of Care #2*
Mood state	☑	☐	*Plan of Care #2*
Behavior problem	☑	☐	*Plan of Care #5*
Activities	☑	☐	*Plan of Care #1*
Falls	☑	☐	*Plan of Care #6*
Nutritional status	☑	☐	*Plan of Care #1*
Feeding tubes	☐	☑	*N/A See dietary note 11/2/91*
Dehydration and fluid maintenance	☐	☑	*Plan of Care #6*
Dental care	☑	☐	*Plan of Care #3*
Pressure ulcers	☑	☐	*Plan of Care #9*
Psychotroplc drug use	☐	☑	*N/A See neuro note 11/2/91*
Physical restraints	☑	☐	*Plan of Care #1*

> Note the care plan number.

> This form identifies patient problems. . .

> . . .and the existence of a corresponding plan of care.

PASARR form. (See *Preadmission Screening Annual Resident Review form,* page 168.)

Initial nursing assessment

This required form is similar to the initial assessment form used in other settings. When documenting your initial assessment in a long-term care setting, place special emphasis on the patient's:
- activity level
- hearing and vision
- bowel and bladder control
- ability to communicate
- safety
- need for adaptive devices to assist dexterity and mobility
- family relationships
- transition from home or hospital to the long-term care facility.

Nursing summaries

Care and status updates must be completed regularly in long-term care facilities. Usually, you must complete a standard nursing care summary at least once every 2 to 4 weeks for patients with specific problems (such as pressure ulcers) who are receiving skilled care. A summary addressing the specific problems must be done weekly. For patients receiving intermediate care, a standard nursing care summary is usually required every 2 weeks.

Summing it up

The nursing summary describes the following:
- patient's ability to perform ADLs
- nutrition and hydration
- safety measures, such as bed rails, restraints, or adaptive devices
- medications and other treatments
- any problems the patient has adjusting to the long-term care facility.

In addition, you must complete a nursing assessment summary at least monthly to comply with Medicare and Medicaid standards.

(Text continues on page 174.)

> *Art of the chart*

Preadmission Screening Annual Resident Review form

Before a patient covered by Medicare or Medicaid enters a long-term care facility, he must undergo an evaluation of mental status, using the Preadmission Screening Annual Resident Review (PASARR). This form is shown below.

PREADMISSION SCREENING ANNUAL RESIDENT REVIEW (PASARR)
IDENTIFICATION FORM PA-PASARR-ID

Applicant's/resident's name - Last, First	Social security number	Date
Vogel, John	*012-34-5678*	*11/10/91*

I.   What are the applicant's/resident's current diagnoses? The individual named above is being considered for nursing facility services on the basis of the following medical diagnoses (Dx).

Primary Dx	(R) *below the knee amputation*
Secondary Dx	*NIDDM - non-insulin dependent diabetes mellitus*
Dx	*Depression*

> **If the patient is diagnosed as having a serious mental disorder, document the diagnosis here.**

individual is considered to have a serious mental illness (MI) if he/she meets all of the following requirements regarding agnosis, level of impairment, and duration of illness.

Diagnosis: The individual has a serious mental disorder diagnosable under the Diagnostic and Statistical Manual of Mental Disorders, 4th edition, revised in 1994.

This mental disorder is:

schizophrenia, delusional (paranoid) disorder, mood disorder, or psychotic disorder not otherwise specified; panic or other severe anxiety disorder; somatoform disorder; personality disorder; or another mental disorder that may lead to a chronic disability. Specify: _*Depression*_

NOTE: For this purpose, individuals whose primary diagnosis is not considered a serious mental illness and who have a diagnosis of dementia (including Alzheimer's disease and other organic brain diseases) are to be excluded from PASARR evaluation and continue with regular admission.

☑ Yes   ☐ No

B.   **Level of impairment:** The mental disorder resulted in functional limitations in major life activities within the past 3 to 6 months that were not appropriate for the individual's developmental stage. An individual typically has at least one of the following characteristics on a continuing or intermittent basis. Check the appropriate box(es):

☑ 1.   Interpersonal functioning. The individual has serious difficulty interacting appropriately and communicating effectively with other individuals, has a possible history of altercations, evictions, firing, fear of strangers, avoidance of interpersonal relationships, and social isolation.

☑ 2.   Concentration, persistence, and pace. The individual has serious difficulty in sustaining focused attention for a long enough period to permit the completion of tasks commonly found in work settings or in worklike structured activities occurring in school or home settings. This manifests difficulties in concentration, inability to complete simple tasks within an established time period, making frequent errors, or requiring assistance in the completion of these tasks.

☑ 3.   Adaptation to change. The individual has serious difficulty in adapting to typical changes in circumstances associated with work, school, family, or social interaction. This manifests in agitation, exacerbated signs and symptoms associated with the illness, or withdrawal from the situation, or requires intervention by the mental health or judicial system.

> **This section asks you to identify the patient's level of impairment—important information for developing a plan of care.**

Preadmission Screening Annual Resident Review form *(continued)*

Completing questions about mental status allows for further evaluation and treatment, if necessary.

Name of prior treatment facility.

Remember, also, that assessment of mental status is a JCAHO requirement.

C. **Recent treatment:** The treatment history indicates that the individual has experienced at least one of the following (check the appropriate boxes):

   1. Psychiatric treatment more intensive than outpatient psychiatric care more than once in the past 2 years (such as partial hospitalization or inpatient hospitalization). Name of inpatient facility partial program or other treatment: *Suburban Hospital*

☑ 2. Within the last 2 years, due to his mental disorder, the individual experienced an episode of significant disruption to the normal living situation, for which supportive services were required to maintain functioning at home, or in a residential treatment environment, or which resulted in intervention by housing or law enforcement officials.

D. Does the applicant/resident meet all of the requirements of having a serious mental illness listed in Section II A-C?

   ☑ Yes   ☐ No

III. An applicant/resident is considered to be mentally retarded if all of the criteria listed below in A through C are met. If evidence is not present to at least suspect that the individual meets each of the three criteria, the individual should not be identified within the mental retardation target population. Documentation is not necessary to support each criterion as long as the individual is suspected to meet each criterion based on observations and knowledge about the individual. The individual completing this form is responsible for reporting the documentation used in making the identification and should complete the entire section, including "Related Questions."

A. The individual has significantly subaverage intellectual functioning (i.e., two standard deviations below the norm, an I.Q. of around 70 or below).

   ☐ Yes   ☐ No

Related Questions:

Is intellectual functioning documented on a standardized general intelligence test?

   ☐ Yes   ☐ No

If yes, what is the name and date of the test and the tester's professional qualifications?

_____

_____

_____

_____

If no, what is the basis of the reviewer's finding?

_____

_____

_____

_____

B. The individual has impairments in adaptive behavior that show (check all that apply):

   ☐ 1. Significant limitation in meeting the standards of maturation, learning, personal independence, and/or social responsibility of his/her age and cultural group.

(continued)

Preadmission Screening Annual Resident Review form (continued)

> Assessing the patient's functional limitations enables you to formulate a plan to promote the highest level of functioning.

☐ 2. Substantial functional limitation in three or more of the following areas of major life activity which is not related to the normal aging process (check all that apply):

☐ a. Self-care　　☐ b. Receptive and expressive language　　☐ c. Learning

☐ d. Mobility　　☐ e. Self-direction　　☐ f. Capacity for independent living

☐ g. Economic self-sufficiency

Related Questions:

Are impairments in adaptive behavior documented by a standardized test?

☐ Yes　　☐ No

If yes, what is the name and date of the test and the tester's professional qualifications?

_____

_____

If no, what is the basis for the reviewer's finding?

_____

_____

C. Is there documentation to substantiate that these conditions occurred between the individual's birth and 22nd birthday?

☐ Yes　　☐ No

Related Questions:

What documentation substantiates that these conditions occurred between the individual's birth and 22nd birthday?

_____

_____

_____

D. Does the applicant/resident have presenting evidence to indicate mental retardation based on the criteria listed in A through C above?

☐ Yes　　☑ No

E. Has the applicant/resident received mental retardation services from an MR agency in the past?

☐ Yes　　Identify agency: _____

☑ No

IV. "Other related condition" (ORC) includes physical, sensory, or neurologic disabilities that manifested before age 22, are likely to continue indefinitely, and result in substantial functional limitations in three or more of the following areas of major life activity: economic self-sufficiency, capacity for independent living, mobility, self-direction, learning, understanding and use of language, and self-care. Examples of individuals with other related conditions include individuals with paraplegia or quadriplegia (due to spinal cord injuries), spina bifida, cerebral palsy, blindness/deafness, epilepsy, head injuries or other injuries (such as gunshot wounds), so long as the injuries were sustained before age 22. It is important to note that an individual can have an ORC regardless of whether the ORC impairs his intellectual abilities.

Preadmission Screening Annual Resident Review form *(continued)*

> Assessing for other related conditions helps to avoid misinterpretation of the patient's status.

The key to determining whether an individual has an ORC is the age of onset of the disability. It's the obligation of the nursing facility to determine age of onset. If the clinical record does not clearly eliminate the possibility that the individual's physical disability occurred before the age of 22, the nursing facility must ask the individual (or the individual's family if necessary), document the response, and target the individual accordingly. This information must be available upon request to representatives of the Department, which include the Community Services Program for Persons with Physical Disabilities (CSPPPD) contractors who serve individuals with other related conditions.

A. An individual is considered to have an ORC, which is a severe chronic developmental disability, if he meets all of the conditions in 1 through 4 below.

> This section identifies other related conditions.

1. The ORC is attributable to:

   a. Cerebral palsy, autism, epilepsy, Tourette syndrome, meningitis, encephalitis, hydrocephalus, multiple sclerosis, polio, anoxic brain damage, paraplegia or quadriplegia (due to spinal cord injuries), spina bifida, blindness or deafness, head injuries, or other injuries (such as gunshot wounds), as long as the injuries were sustained before age 22. Circle applicable condition(s).

   b. Any other condition, other than a serious mental illness, found to be closely related to mental retardation because this condition has resulted in impairment of general intellectual functioning or adaptive behavior similar to that of individuals with mental retardation, and requires treatment or services similar to those required for individuals with mental retardation.

2. The ORC is manifested before the individual reaches age 22.

3. The ORC is likely to continue indefinitely.

4. The ORC results in substantial functional limitations in three or more of the following areas of major life activity. Check all areas of substantial functional limitation that were present prior to age 22 and were directly the result of the other related condition:

   ☐ a. Self-care   ☐ b. Understanding and use of language   ☐ c. Learning

   ☐ d. Mobility   ☐ e. Self-direction   ☐ f. Capacity for independent living

   ☐ g. Economic self-sufficiency

B. Does the applicant/resident meet the criteria of an ORC as defined in IV-A?

   ☐ Yes   ☑ No

C. Is there documentation that indicates the presence of an ORC as defined in IV-A?

   ☐ Yes   ☑ No

D. Was the individual referred for care by an agency that serves individuals with developmental disabilities or is the applicant/resident eligible for that agency's services?

   ☐ Yes   ☑ No

IF YOU ANSWER "YES" IN SECTIONS II-D (MH), III-D (MR), OR IV-B (ORC) - GO TO SECTION V.

IF YOU ANSWER "NO" IN SECTIONS II-D (MH), III-D (MR) AND IV-B (ORC) - GO TO SECTION VI-A-B.

(continued)

Preadmission Screening Annual Resident Review form *(continued)*

V. Does the applicant/resident meet the criteria for exceptional admission to a facility without PAS evaluation?

Criteria defined in A, B, and C of this section apply to applicants/residents who answered "Yes" in Sections II-D, IV-B.

A. Is person an exempted hospital discharge?

     ☑ Yes   ☐ No

> A patient admitted directly from a hospital may be allowed to stay in a long-term care facility for 30 days without further evaluation.

Although identified as an individual with a serious mental illness, mental retardation, or an ORC, an applicant/resident who is not dangerous to himself and/or others may be directly admitted for nursing facility services from an acute care hospital for a period up to 30 days without further evaluation if such admission is based on a written, medically prescribed period of recovery for the conditions requiring hospitalization.

If the individual is admitted under this criteria and continues in residence for more than 30 days, a new PA-PASARR-ID form must be completed. The Department must be notified on the MA 408, and an evaluation must be completed within 40 calendar days of admission to the nursing facility. Failure to report these changes in condition in a timely manner may result in financial sanctions against the nursing facility.

B. Does person require respite care?

     ☐ Yes   ☐ No

Although identified as an individual with a serious* mental illness, mental retardation, or other related condition, an applicant/resident who is not dangerous to self or others may be admitted for respite care for a period up to 14 days without further evaluation if he or she is certified by a referring or attending physician to require 24-hour nursing facility services and supervision.

If the individual's condition changes from respite to long-term and he/she is going to stay in the nursing facility, the department must be notified on the MA 408, and an evaluation must be completed within 24 days of admission to the nursing facility. Failure to report these changes in condition in a timely manner may result in financial sanctions against the nursing facility.

C. Is person in a coma or functioning at brain stem level?

     ☐ Yes   ☐ No

Although identified as an individual with a serious* mental illness, mental retardation, or other related condition, an applicant/resident who is not dangerous to himself and/or others may receive nursing facility services without further evaluation if certified by the referring or attending physician to be in a coma or functioning at brain stem level. The condition must require intense 24-hour nursing facility services and supervision and is so extreme that the individual cannot focus upon, participate in, or benefit from specialized services.

If there is a "No" response in Sections II-D, III-D, and IV-B, complete Section VI A-B.

If there is a "Yes" response in Sections II-D (MH), III-D (MR), or IV-B(ORC), and if all answers to Section V (Exceptional criteria) are "No," complete Sections VI-A and VI-C.

If there is a "Yes" response to any question in Section V (Exceptional criteria), complete Sections VI-A and VI-D.

*Serious only applies to mental illness

VI. Certifications

A. Individual Completing Form:

     Cindy Graham, MSW   *(210) 555-1111*   *11/11/91*
     SIGNATURE   TELEPHONE NUMBER   DATE

> Signature, date, and phone number.

Preadmission Screening Annual Resident Review form *(continued)*

> Whether or not further evaluation is needed depends on answers to previous questions.

GO TO APPROPRIATE BLOCK: B. C. OR D.

B. Regular Admission - No further PASARR evaluation is needed. (Answers in Sections II-D, III-D, AND IV-B are all "No".) This is to certify that the applicant does not need to have a PASARR evaluation completed.

_____
SIGNATURE   TELEPHONE NUMBER   DATE

GO TO SECTION VII

C. Target Group - PASARR evaluation is required. (Answers in Sections II-D, III-D, or IV-B are "Yes" and answers to Section V are "No"'.) This is to certify that the applicant meets criteria for referral to the designated Area Agency on Aging for PAS evaluation or if a resident will be referred to the Department's Utilization Management Review Team for PASARR evaluation.

_____
SIGNATURE   TELEPHONE NUMBER   DATE

GO TO SECTION VII

D. Exceptional Admission (when answers in Sections II-D, III-D, or IV-B are "Yes" and one or more answers in Section V is "Yes"). This is to certify that the applicant/resident was targeted for evaluation but has a condition that meets the criteria for exceptional admission indicated in Section V.

Dr. Steven Humbert   *(210) 555-1234*
PRINT PHYSICIAN'S NAME   TELEPHONE NUMBER

Dr. Steven Humbert
PHYSICIAN'S SIGNATURE   DATE

Medical Director Confirmation (must be completed for all exceptional admissions)

This is to confirm that I have reviewed the diagnosis and medical need of the applicant for the level of nursing services and medical services to be provided by the facility.

Dr. Louise McCarthy   *(210) 555-9816*
PRINT MEDICAL DIRECTOR'S NAME   TELEPHONE NUMBER

Dr. Louise McCarthy
MEDICAL DIRECTOR'S SIGNATURE   DATE

GO TO SECTION VII

/II. Does the applicant/resident need an interpreter or other assistance to participate in or understand the PASARR evaluation process?

    ☐ Yes   Describe: _____
    ☑ No

GO TO SECTION VIII

/III. Type of Admission

    ☐ Target group   ☑ Exceptional admission   ☐ Regular

        1. Report on MA 408   1. Report on MA 408 admission

        2. Refer to OPTIONS/UMR team

ADL checklists and flow sheets

ADL checklists and flow sheets are standard forms that are usually completed by a nursing assistant on each shift; then you review and sign them. These forms tell the health care team members about the patient's abilities, degree of independence, and special needs so they can determine the type of assistance each patient requires.

The following tools will help you assess and document ADLs:
- Katz index
- Lawton scale
- Barthel index and scale.

Katz index

The Katz index ranks the patient's ability in six areas:

    bathing

    dressing

    toileting

    moving from wheelchair to bed and returning

    continence

    feeding.

It describes his functional level at a specific time and rates his performance of each function on three levels: performing without help, needing some help, or having complete disability. (See *Rating ability to perform basic tasks*.)

Lawton scale

The Lawton scale evaluates the patient's ability to perform complex personal care activities necessary for independent living. Activities include:
- using the telephone
- cooking
- shopping
- doing laundry
- managing finances
- taking medications
- preparing meals.

Activities are rated on a three-point scale, ranging from without help (3), to needing some help (2), to com-

Art of the chart

Rating ability to perform basic tasks

The Katz index, shown below, is used to assess six basic ADLs.

Resident's name and the date

Evaluation Form

Name _Henry Dancer_ Date _12/4/91_

For each area of functioning listed below, check the description that applies. (The word "assistance" means supervision, direction, or personal assistance.)

Bathing: Sponge bath, tub bath, or shower.

☐ Receives no assistance; gets into and out of tub, if tub is usual means of bathing.

☑ Receives assistance in bathing only one part of the body, such as the back or leg.

◯ Receives assistance in bathing more than one part of the body, or can't bathe.

The focus of this chart is on basic activities.

Dressing: Gets outer garments and underwear from closets and drawers and uses fasteners, including suspenders, if worn.

☐ Gets clothes and gets completely dressed without assistance.

☐ Gets clothes and gets dressed without assistance except for tying shoes.

☑ Receives assistance in getting clothes or in getting dresses, or stays partly or completely undressed.

Toileting: Goes to the room termed "toilet" for bowel movement and urination, cleans self afterward, and arranges clothes.

☐ Goes to toilet room, cleans self, and arranges clothes without assistance. May use object for support, such as cane, walker, or wheelchair and may manage night bedpan or commode, emptying it in the morning.

☑ Receives assistance in going to toilet room or in cleaning self or arranging clothes after elimination or in use of night bedpan or commode.

◯ Doesn't go to toilet room for the elimination process.

Transfer

☐ Moves into and out of bed and chair without assistance. May use object, such as cane or walker for support.

☑ Moves into or out of bed or chair with assistance.

◯ Doesn't get out of bed.

Continence

☑ Controls urination and bowel movement completely by self.

◯ Has occasional accidents.

◯ Supervision helps keep control of urination or bowel movement, or catheter is used, or is incontinent.

Feeding

☐ Feeds self without assistance.

☑ Feeds self except for assistance in cutting meat or buttering bread.

◯ Receives assistance in feeding or is fed partly or completely through tubes or by I.V. fluids.

Evaluator: _Germaine Fried, RN_

Index

☐ **Indicates independence** ◯ **Indicates dependence**

A: Independent in all six functions.
B: Independent in all but one of these functions.
C: Independent in all but bathing and one additional function.
D: Independent in all but bathing, dressing and one additional function.
E: Independent in all but bathing, dressing, toileting, and one additional function.

F: Independent in all but bathing, dressing, toileting, transferring, and one additional function.
G: Dependent in all six functions.
Other: Dependent in at least two functions but not classifiable as C, D, E, or F.

Adapted with permission from Katz, S. et al. "Studies of Illness in the Aged: The Index of ADL-A Standardized Measure of Biological and Psychosocial Function," *JAMA* 185:914-19, ©1993, American Medical Association

plete disability (1). (See *Rating ability to perform complex tasks.*)

Barthel index and scale

The Barthel index and scale is used to evaluate:
• feeding
• moving from wheelchair to bed and returning
• performing personal hygiene
• getting on and off the toilet
• bathing
• walking on a level surface or propelling a wheelchair
• going up and down stairs
• dressing and undressing
• maintaining bowel continence
• controlling the bladder.

Each item is scored according to the amount of assistance needed. Over time, results reveal improvement or decline. Another scale, the Barthel Self-Care Rating Scale, evaluates function in more detail. (See *Getting better or worse?* pages 178 and 179.)

Plans of care

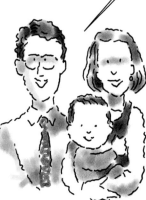

Remember to keep family members involved in your plan of care.

Standards for plans of care are developed by individual long-term care facilities. When a patient is admitted to a facility, an interim plan of care is used until there is an interdisciplinary care conference regarding this patient. After this, a full plan of care is developed for the patient. This plan must be completed by the nurse within 7 days of the patient's admission. A documented review of the plan must be completed every 3 months or when the patient's status changes.

In long-term care settings, plans of care usually evolve from an interdisciplinary approach to care, with contributions by the patient, members of his family, and other health care providers.

As always, base your plan of care on the patient's health problems, the nursing diagnoses, and the expected treatment outcomes. Include measurable patient outcomes with reasonable time frames and specific interventions to achieve them.

(Text continues on page 180.)

Art of the chart

Rating ability to perform complex tasks

The Lawton Scale below provides information about a patient's ability to perform more sophisticated tasks than basic ADLs.

Resident name

Date

Name _John Shapiro_   Rated by _James Mott, RN_   Date _Dec. 12, 1991_

1. Can you use the telephone?
   without help .... Your name ...(3)
   with some help 2
   completely unable 1
2. Can you get to places beyond walking distance?
   without help 3
   with some help .... (2)
   not without special arrangements 1
3. Can you go shopping for groceries?
   without help 3
   with some help .... (2)
   completely unable 1
4. Can you prepare your own meals?
   without help .... (3)
   with some help 2
   completely unable 1
5. Can you do your own housework?
   without help .... (3)
   with some help 2
   completely unable 1
6. Can you do your own handyman work?
   without help 3
   with some help .... (2)
   completely unable 1

7. Can you do your own laundry?
   without help .... (3)
   with some help 2
   completely unable 1
8a. Do you take medicines or use any medications?
   Yes (If yes, answer Question 8b.) .... (1)
   No (If no, answer Question 8c.) 2
8b. Do you take your own medicine?
   without help (in the right doses at the right times) ....(3)
   with some help (if someone prepares it for you and/or re-
   minds you to take it) 2
   completely unable 1
8c. If you had to take medicine, could you do it?
   without help (in the right doses at the right time) 3
   with some help (if someone prepared it for you and/or reminded you to take it) 2
   completely unable 1
9. Can you manage your own money?
   without help .... (3)
   with some help 2
   completely unable 1

Activities are rated on a three-point scale.

Questions may need to be modified for individual patients.

The first answer in each case—except for 8a—indicates independence; the second indicates capability with as-sistance; and the third, dependence. In this version the maximum score is 29, although scores have meaning only for a particular patient, as when declining scores over time reveal deterioration.

Adapted with permission from Lawton, M.P., and Brody, E.M., "Assessment of Older People: Self-Maintaining and Instrumental Activities of Daily Living," *The Gerontologist* 9(3):179-186, Autumn 1969.

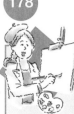

Art of the chart

Getting better or worse?

The Barthel index shown below is used to assess the patient's ability to perform 10 activities of daily living, document findings for other health care team members, and reveal improvement or decline.

Date _December 14, 1991_

Patient's name _Jack Boyd_

Evaluator _Kate Roth, RN_

Action	With help	Independent
Feeding (if food needs to be cut up = help)	5	(10)
Moving from wheelchair to bed and return (includes sitting up in bed)	5 to (10)	15
Personal toilet (wash face, comb hair, shave, clean teeth)	0	(5)
Getting on and off toilet (handling clothes, wipe, flush)	(5)	10
Bathing self	0	(5)
Walking on level surface (or, if unable to walk, propelling wheelchair)	0	(5) or 15
Ascending and descending stairs	(5)	10
Dressing (includes tying shoes, fastening fasteners)	(5)	10
Controlling bowels	5	(10)
Controlling bladder	(5)	10

Definition and Discussion of Scoring

A person scoring 100 is continent, feeds himself, dresses ⸺⸺⸺⸺ and chairs, bathes himself, walks at least a block, and can ascend and descend stairs. This doesn't ⸺⸺⸺⸺ one; he may not be able to cook, keep house, or meet the public, but he's able to get along without atte⸺⸺

> Reading the definitions of the numbers will enable you to interpret the scale.

Feeding

10 = Independent. The person can feed himself a mea⸺⸺⸺⸺ omeone puts the food within his reach. He must be able to put on an assistive dev⸺⸺ if needed, ⸺⸺⸺⸺ alt and pepper, spread butter, and so forth. Also, he must accomplish these tasks in a reasonable time.

5 = The person needs some help with cutting up food and other tasks, as listed above.

Moving from wheelchair to bed and return

15 = The person operates independently in all phases of this activity. He can safely approach the bed in his wheelchair, lock brakes, lift footrests, move safely from bed, lie down, come to a sitting position on the side of the bed, change the position of the wheelchair, if necessary, to transfer back into it safely, and return to the wheelchair.

10 = Either the person needs some minimal help in some step of this activity, or needs to be reminded or supervised for safety in one or more parts of this activity.

5 = The person can come to a sitting position without the help of a second person but needs to be lifted out of bed, or needs a great deal of help with transfers.

Handling personal toilet

5 = The person can wash hands and face, comb hair, clean teeth, and shave. He may use any kind of razor but he must be able to get it from the drawer or cabinet and plug it in or put in a blade without help. A female must put on her own makeup, if any, but need not braid or style her hair.

Getting better or worse? *(continued)*

Getting on and off toilet
10 = The person is able to get on and off the toilet, unfasten and refasten clothes, prevent soiling of clothes, and use toilet paper without help. He may use a wall bar or other stable object for support, if needed. If he needs to use a bed pan instead of toilet, he must be able to place it on a chair, use it competently, and empty and clean it.
5 = The person needs help to overcome imbalance, handle clothes, or use toilet paper.
Bathing self
5 = The person may use a bath tub or shower or give himself a complete sponge bath. Regardless of method, he must be able to complete all the steps involved without another person's presence.
Walking on a level surface
15 = The person can walk at least 50 yards without help or supervision. He may wear braces or prostheses and use crutches, canes, or a walkerette, but not a rolling walker. He must be able to lock and unlock braces, if used, get the necessary mechanical aids into position for use, stand up and sit down, and dispose of the aids when he sits. (Putting on, fastening, and taking off braces is scored under Dressing).
5 = If the person can't ambulate but can propel a wheelchair independently, he must be able to go around corners, turn around, maneuver the chair to table, bed, toilet, and other locations. He must be able to push a chair at least 150' (45.7 m). Don't score this item if the person receives a score for walking.
0 = unable to walk
Ascending and descending stairs
10 = The person can go up and down a flight of stairs safely without help or supervision. He may and should use handrails, canes, or crutches when needed, and he must be able to carry canes or crutches as he ascends or descends.
5 = The person needs help with or supervision of any one of the above items.
Dressing and undressing
10 = The person can put on, fasten, and remove all clothing (including any prescribed corset or braces) and tie shoe laces (unless he requires adaptations for this). Such special clothing as suspenders, loafers, and dresses that open down the front may be used when necessary.
5 = The person needs help in putting on, fastening, or removing any clothing. He must do at least half the work himself and must accomplish the task in a reasonable time. Women need not be scored on use of a brassiere or girdle unless these are prescribed garments.
Controlling bowels
10 = The person can control his bowels without accidents. He can use a suppository or take an enema when necessary (as in spinal cord injury patients who have had bowel training).
5 = The person needs help in using a suppository or taking an enema or has occasional accidents.
Controlling bladder
10 = The person can control his bladder day and night. Spinal cord injury patients who wear an external device and leg bag must put them on independently, clean and empty the bag, and stay dry, day and night.
5 = The person has occasional accidents, can't wait for the bed pan or get to the toilet in time, or needs help with an external device.

The total score is less significant or meaningful than the individual items, because these indicate where the deficiencies lie. Any applicant to a long-term care facility who scores 100 should be evaluated carefully before admission to see whether admission is indicated. Discharged patients with scores of 100 shouldn't require further physical therapy but may benefit from a home visit to see whether any environmental adjustments are needed.

This scale clearly explains how to rate the patient.

Adapted with permission from Mahoney, F.I. and Barthel, D.W. "Functional Evaluation: The Barthel Index," *Maryland State Medical Journal* 14:62, 1965.

Discharge and transfer forms

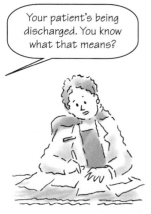

Your patient's being discharged. You know what that means?

When the facility discharges a patient back home or to a hospital, you must document the reason for discharge, the patient's destination, his mode of transportation, and the person or staff member accompanying him, if appropriate.

Other important data to include in this document are a list of prescribed medications, skin assessment findings, overall condition, the disposition of personal belongings, and teaching topics that you covered (regarding diet, medications, skin care, and other areas).

Guidelines drawn up by the Joint Commission on Accreditation of Healthcare Organizations emphasize the need to assess and summarize the patient's condition at transfer time. (See *Transfer and personal belongings form.*)

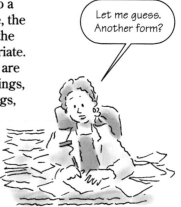

Let me guess. Another form?

Documentation guidelines

In long-term care facilities, consider the following points when updating your records:
• When writing nursing summaries, address specific patient problems noted in the plan of care.
• When writing progress notes, confirm that the patient's progress is being evaluated and reevaluated in relation to the goals or outcomes in the plan of care. If goals aren't met, address this. Also describe and document additional actions.
• Record transfers and discharges according to facility protocol.
• Document changes in the patient's condition and report them to the doctor and the family within 24 hours.
• Document follow-up interventions or other measures taken in response to a change in the patient's condition.
• Keep a record of visits from family or friends and of phone calls about the patient. Your facility may be fined by state or federal regulators if these aren't charted.
• If an incident occurs, such as a fall or a treatment error, fill out an incident report and write follow-up notes for at least 48 hours after the incident (or follow your facility's policy).
• During the patient's first week of residence, keep detailed records on each shift.

Art of the chart

Transfer and personal belongings form

Patients in long-term care facilities may be admitted to the hospital, discharged to home, or transferred to other facilities. The forms below are used during this process.

1. PATIENT'S LAST NAME	FIRST NAME	MI	2. SEX	3. SOCIAL SECURITY NUMBER
Clark	Robert	T	Male	144-44-4444

4. PATIENT'S ADDRESS (Street, City, State, Zip Code) 1 Wise street Springhouse, PA 19477

5. DATE OF BIRTH 2-8-28

6. RELIGION unknown

7. DATE OF THIS TRANSFER 12/29/91

8. FACILITY NAME AND ADDRESS TRANSFERRING TO Seniors Care Facility 22 Elderly Way Phila., PA

9. PHYSICIAN IN CHARGE AT TIME OF TRANSFER Dr. Nicholas
Will this physician care for patient after admission to new facility? ❑ YES ☒ NO

10. DATES OF STAY AT FACILITY TRANSFERRING FROM

ADMISSION 11/14/91   DISCHARGE 12/29/91

11. PAYMENT SOURCE FOR CHARGES TO PATIENT

A. ☒ SELF OR FAMILY
B. ❑ PRIVATE INSURANCE

C. ❑ BLUE CROSS BLUE SHIELD
D. ❑ EMPLOYER OR UNION

E. ❑ PUBLIC AGENCY (Give name)
F. ❑ OTHER (Explain)

12-A. NAME AND ADDRESS OF FACILITY TRANSFERRING FROM Community Hospital   3000 Medical Way, Phila., PA

12-B. NAMES AND ADDRESSES OF ALL HOSPITALS AND EXTENDED CARE FACILITIES FROM WHICH PATIENT WAS DISCHARGED IN PAST 60 DAYS.

13. CLINIC APPOINTMENT   DATE   TIME   CLINIC APPOINTMENT CARD ATTACHED

14. DATE OF LAST PHYSICAL EXAMINATION 12/26/91

15. RELATIVE OR GUARDIAN: Name Katherine Clark   Address 1 Wise street Springhouse, PA 19477   Phone number 1-215-999-9000

16. DIAGNOSES AT TIME OF TRANSFER
(a) Primary ® CVA
(b) Secondary IDDM

EMPLOYMENT RELATED:
❑ YES
☒ NO

VITALS AT TIME OF TRANSFER
T 98° P 68 R 20 B/P 140/82

ADVANCE DIRECTIVES ❑ YES ☒ NO ❑ COPY ATTACHED
CODE STATUS Full code

CHECK ALL THAT APPLY
Disabilities
☒ Speech
❑ Hearing
☒ Vision
❑ Sensation
Incontinence
☒ Bladder
☒ Bowel
☒ Saliva

❑ Amputation
☒ Paralysis (L) side
❑ Contracture
❑ Pressure Ulcer
Impairments
❑ Mental

Activity Tolerance Limitations
❑ None
☒ Moderate
❑ Severe
Patient knows diagnosis?
☒ Yes
❑ No

Potential for Rehabilitation
❑ Good
☒ Fair
❑ Poor
IMPORTANT MEDICAL INFORMATION
(State allergies if any)
PCN

DIET, DRUGS, AND OTHER THERAPY at time of discharge
-Mechanical soft diet (2,000 cal)
-Megace 4 tabs 06h
-Lasix 40 mg P.O. b.i.d.
-Aspirin 81mg P.O. q.d.
-Humabid 7½ 20 units q.a.m. & h.s.
-Sliding scale coverage BS <40 7400
-Call Dr. Nicholas, BS 200-250:2u | 301-350:4u
   251-300:3u | 351-400:5u   } Humulin R
(Physician, please sign below)

SUGGESTIONS FOR ACTIVE CARE
BED
Position in good body alignment and change position every 2 hrs.
Avoid flat supine position
Prone position 2 time/day as tolerated.
SITTING
4 hr 3 times/day

WEIGHT BEARING
❑ Full
☒ Partial
❑ None
on _____ Leg

EXERCISES
Range of motion 3 times/day.
to (L) extremities by
❑ patient ❑ nurse ❑ family
Stand 3 min. 2 times/day.

LOCOMOTION
Walk unable times/day.
SOCIAL ACTIVITIES
Encourage (☒ Group ❑ Individual) activities (☒ within ❑ outside) home.
❑ Transportation: ☒ Ambulance
❑ Car ❑ Car for handicapped
❑ Bus

Signature of Physician or Nurse John Brown, RN   Date 12 / 29 / 91

Transfer and personal belongings form (continued)

Any articles of clothing or other belongings left at the hospital will be held for 30 days after discharge. Items remaining after this period will be disposed of by the hospital.

			COMMENTS
Date: 12/29/91			
Initials: CR			
VALUABLES DESCRIBE			
Wallet:		✓	1 brown leather wallet
Money (Amount): $25.00		✓	1-$20.00 bill 5 $1 bills
Watch:			
Jewelry:			
Glasses/Contacts: Glasses		✓	Wire rim-gold
Hearing Aids:			
Dentures:		✓	
Partial			
Complete		✓	Container labeled
Keys			
ARTICLE DESCRIBE			
Ambulatory Aids:			
Cane, Walker, Etc.			
Bedclothes		✓	1 pair plaid pajamas
Belt			
Dress			
Outer Wear			
Pants			
Pocketbook			
Shirt			
Shoes			
Sweater			
Undergarments			
Other			

All belongings were sent home with patient's family: YES   (NO)

Patient's Signature ___Bob Clark_____

Witnessed by Hospital Personnel ___Mary Jones, RN_____

• Flag a new patient by putting a red dot on the chart, bed, or door or by using a similar system, so that all staff members are aware of the new resident and become familiar with him. (Remember to be sensitive to each patient's need for confidentiality and dignity, however.)

• Keep reimbursement in mind when documenting. For a facility to qualify for payment, its records must clearly reflect the level of care given to the patient.

• Be sure that your records accurately reflect skilled services that the patient receives.

• Always record a doctor's verbal and telephone orders and have the doctor countersign them within 48 hours.

• Document visits by the doctor to the patient. Generally accepted standards require one visit after admission, another after the first 30 days, and at least one every 60 days thereafter.

> Had enough documentation? Well then, take our quick quiz.

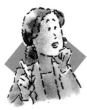

Quick quiz

1. The two levels of care in long-term care settings are:
A. skilled and intermediate.
B. acute and critical.
C. geriatric and special need.

Answer: A. Skilled and intermediate care differ in the amount and type of nursing skills provided.

2. The MDS is required by:
A. Medicare.
B. Medicaid.
C. OBRA.

Answer: C. Under the federal law known as OBRA, an initial assessment must be documented on an MDS form.

3. In a long-term care facility, you must write a plan of care within:
A. 14 days of the patient's admission.
B. 7 hours of the patient's admission.
C. 7 days of the patient's admission.

Answer: C. You must complete the plan of care within 7 days of admission and update and review it every 3 months.

4. A tool for assessing the patient's mental status is:

    A. the Katz index.

    B. the Lawton scale.

    C. the PASARR form.

Answer: C. A PASARR, or Preadmission Screening Annual Resident Review, form is required by Medicare and Medicaid for reimbursement.

5. Medicare and Medicaid require nursing assessment summaries to be completed:

    A. weekly.

    B. monthly.

    C. daily.

Answer: B. In addition, nursing care summaries must be completed at least once a week for patients receiving skilled care and every 2 weeks for those receiving intermediate care.

6. Patients in a long-term facility must be seen by the doctor:

    A. at least once every 60 days.

    B. at least once a month.

    C. at least once every 6 months.

Answer: A. Patients are seen by doctors on an as-needed basis, but they must be seen at least every 60 days.

Scoring

☆☆☆   If you answered all six items correctly, outasight! You're PASARR (Perfectly Amazing, Stupendous, and Artful at Records and Reports)!

☆☆   If you answered four or five correctly, unreal! No doubt about it, you're the RAP (Really Awesome Paperwork) expert!

☆   If you answered fewer than four correctly, keep plugging! You're an ADL (Admirably Dedicated Learner).

Part III

Special topics

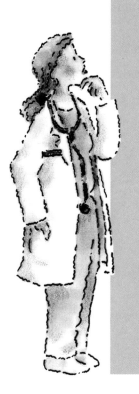

Enhancing your charting

Just the facts

In this chapter, you'll learn:

♦ the seven rules of clear charting and how to follow them

♦ different types of doctors' orders and how to clarify them.

A look at expert charting

Charting like a pro requires adherence to these seven fundamental rules:

Document care completely, concisely, and accurately.

Record observations objectively.

Document information promptly.

Write legibly.

Use approved abbreviations.

Use the proper technique to correct written errors.

Sign all documents as required.

Following these rules enhances communication between all members of the health care team and ensures reimbursement for your facility.

Charting completely, concisely, and accurately

Here are a few quick tips for expressing yourself completely, concisely, and accurately:

- Write clear sentences that get right to the point.
- Don't use long words when short ones will do.
- Clearly identify the subject of each sentence.
- Don't be afraid to use the word "I."

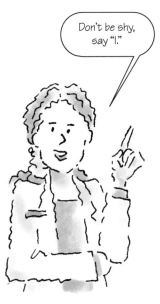

Don't be shy, say "I."

Without these tips, a rambling, vague, and ultimately meaningless note might be written such as *Communication with patient's home initiated today to delineate progression of disease process and describe course of action.* That's mind-boggling.

Instead, put the above tips to work for you, and your charting savvy will shine. Here's how this note should be written: *I contacted Andrea Sovak's daughter by phone at 1300 hours; I explained that Mrs. Sovak's respiratory status had worsened and that she would be moved to the ICU for monitoring.* This clearly differentiates your actions from those of the patient, doctor, or other staff member. (See *Tell it like it is.*)

Don't be wishy-washy

Because we are taught that nurses don't make diagnoses, many of us qualify our observations with words like "ap-

---

Art of the chart

Tell it like it is

In the examples below, the first is incomplete, leaving the reader wondering what really happened. The second is both complete and precise.

The wrong way

Not clear who this is

Date	Time	Sign entries
1/20/91	0200	*Patient deceased at 0150. Next of kin notified.* ———————— *Ann Pine, RN*
1/20/91	0150	*Patient pronounced dead by Dr. Ted Burns.* ———————— *Ann Pine, RN*
1/20/91	0155	*Dr. Ted Burns notified Mary Ritt, sister of patient, of patient's death, by phone.* ——— *Ann Pine, RN*

The right way

Vague wording

This concisely states what occurred.

This clearly states who was notified and by whom.

pears" or "apparently." But using vague language in a patient's chart tells the reader that you aren't sure what you're describing or doing. The right approach is to clearly and succinctly describe what occurred without sounding tentative.

Maintaining objectivity

Knowing what to chart is important, too. Record just the facts — exactly what you see, hear, and do—not your opinions or assumptions. Chart only relevant information relating to patient care and reflecting the nursing process.

Don't put words in other people's mouths

Avoid subjective statements like, *Patient's level of co-operation has deteriorated since yesterday.* Instead, use the patient's exact words to describe the facts that led you to this conclusion. You might write: *The patient stated, "I don't want to learn how to inject insulin. I tried yesterday, but I'm not going to do it today."* (See *Quotations are key.*)

Stick to the facts, leave out opinions; that's my job.

You may also want to chart your subjective conclusion about the patient's condition. That's okay, as long as you also record the objective assessment data that supports it. For example, *Pt sad and tearful with flat affect; states "I miss my family."*

Second-hand data

Document only data that you collect or observe yourself or data from a reliable source, such as the patient or another nurse. When you include data reported by someone else, always cite your source. For example, you may write, *Nurse Ray found pt attempting to climb OOB, pt restrained for safety per hospital protocol.*

Ensuring timeliness

Timely charting includes these essentials:
• charting as soon as possible
• noting exact times
• charting chronologically
• handling late entries correctly.

Art of the chart

Quotations are key

Using the patient's exact words makes your charting accurate and objective. The notes below show how.

> Use the patient's own words as much as possible.

> Special instructions are documented precisely.

> Here's proof of patient teaching.

Date	Time	Sign entries
12/10/91	1300	Pt states she has been voiding drops of bloody urine every 5 to 10 minutes for the last hour. She states she feels "pressure" and a "burning pain" with voiding. Dr. Jones was called. Dr. Jones's answering service responded. Dr. Jones will call back. ——— Tina Clark, RN
12/10/91	1310	Dr. Jones returned call; was informed of pt's symptoms. Order given for Bactrim DS, one, P.O. now and Pyridium 200 mg P.O. now. Will see pt this afternoon. ——— Tina Clark, RN
12/10/91	1320	Bactrim DS, one p.o. and Pyridium 200 mg P.O. given. ——— Tina Clark, RN
12/10/91	1320	I gave pt instructions regarding medication uses and adverse effects; encouraged her to drink plenty of fluids; I explained that Pyridium may stain clothing, turn urine orange-red, and stain contact lenses. ——— Tina Clark, RN
12/10/91	1420	Pt states she has no pain with voiding and that "pressure is also gone." ——— Tina Clark, RN

Chart ASAP

Record information on the patient's chart as soon as possible after you make an observation or provide care. Information charted immediately is more likely to be accurate and complete. If you leave your charting until the end of the shift, you might forget important details.

One way to chart on time is by keeping charting materials at the patient's bedside. But this system can threaten confidentiality. (See *Keeping it confidential,* page 190.)

Give them the time of day

Be specific about times in your charting, especially the exact time of sudden changes in the patient's condition, significant events, and nursing actions. Don't chart in blocks of time, such as *0700 to 1500*. This looks vague, implies inattention to the patient, and makes it hard to determine when specific events occurred. (See *Marking time.*)

Most facilities require nurses to chart in military time, which expresses time as 24 one-hour-long periods per day, rather than 2 sets of 12 one-hour periods. (See *Time marches on.*)

Put your chart in order

Most assessments and observations are useful only as parts of a whole picture. Isolated assessments reveal very little, but in chronological order, they tell the patient's story over time and reveal a pattern of improvement or deterioration.

Charting in chronological order is easy if you jot down your observations and assessments when they occur. Too often, though, nurses wait until the end of a shift, then record groups of assessments that fail to accurately reflect variations in the patient's condition over time. (See *Correct and chronological*, page 192.)

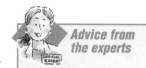

Advice from the experts

Keeping it confidential

Bedside computers are the ultimate in easy charting, and bedside flow sheets or progress notes run a close second. But some nurses feel uncomfortable leaving patient information in full view. Although flow sheets usually don't contain confidential information, progress notes do.

One solution is to keep confidential records in a fold-down desk outside the patient's room. Having a handy writing surface also makes it easier to chart promptly. If your facility doesn't use bedside forms or computers, keep a worksheet or pad in your pocket for note-keeping. Just jot down key phrases and times, then transcribe the information onto the chart later.

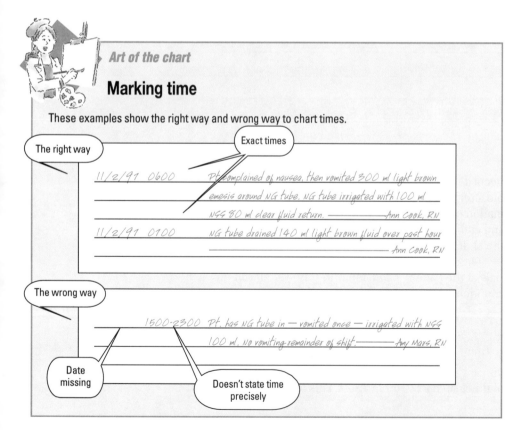

Art of the chart

Marking time

These examples show the right way and wrong way to chart times.

The right way

Exact times

| 11/2/91 | 0600 | Pt. complained of nausea, then vomited 300 ml light brown emesis around NG tube. NG tube irrigated with 100 ml NSS 80 ml clear fluid return. ————————Ann Cook, RN |
| 11/2/91 | 0100 | NG tube drained 140 ml light brown fluid over past hour ————————Ann Cook, RN |

The wrong way

| 1500-2300 | Pt. has NG tube in — vomited once — irrigated with NSS 100 ml. No vomiting-remainder of shift.————Amy Mars, RN |

Date missing

Doesn't state time precisely

Time marches on

Many facilities use military time because it alleviates confusion over a.m. and p.m. entries. Here's how it works:

0100 hours = 1 a.m.		1300 hours = 1 p.m.	
0200 hours = 2 a.m.		1400 hours = 2 p.m.	
0300 hours = 3 a.m.		1500 hours = 3 p.m.	
0400 hours = 4 a.m.		1600 hours = 4 p.m.	
0500 hours = 5 a.m.		1700 hours = 5 p.m.	
0600 hours = 6 a.m.		1800 hours = 6 p.m.	
0700 hours = 7 a.m.		1900 hours = 7 p.m.	
0800 hours = 8 a.m.		2000 hours = 8 p.m.	
0900 hours = 9 a.m.		2100 hours = 9 p.m.	
1000 hours = 10 a.m.		2200 hours = 10 p.m.	
1100 hours = 11 a.m.		2300 hours = 11 p.m.	
1200 hours = 12 noon		2400 hours = 12 midnight	

Better late than never

You may occasionally need to add a late entry in certain situations, such as:
- when the chart is unavailable at the time of the event
- if you forgot to document something
- if you need to add important information.

Bear in mind, though, that late entries can look suspicious during a malpractice trial. Find out if your facility has a protocol for late entries. If not, add the entry on the first available line, and label it *late entry* to indicate that it's out of sequence. Then record the date and time of the entry as well as the date and time when the entry should have been made.

Ensuring legibility

One of the main reasons to document your nursing care is to communicate with other members of the health care team. Trying to decipher sloppy handwriting wastes people's time and puts the patient in jeopardy if critical information is misinterpreted. (See *Neatness counts!* page 193.)

Use printing instead of cursive writing because it's usually easier to understand. If you don't have room to chart something legibly, leave that section blank, put a

Art of the chart

Correct and chronological

Here's an example of charting that's done correctly in chronological order

0800	Neuro: Pt AAO x 3, follows commands, moves all extremities, speech clear and appropriate. Jane Klass, RN
	CV: Afebrile, skin warm, dry and intact, ⊕ palpable pulses no edema. ————————— Jane Klass, RN
	Resp: Bilateral breath sounds, no SOB lungs clear, on room air. ————————— Jane Klass, RN
	Pt complaining of sudden shortness of breath, O₂ 2 L/minute applied, stat chest X-ray obtained, MD notified.
	————————— Jane Klass, RN
0920	Lasix 40 mg I.V. provided to pt. ————————— Jane Klass, RN
0930	Shortness of breath continues, pulse ox 81%, O₂ ↑ to 50% face mask. ————————— Jane Klass, RN
0935	Pt transferred to ICU, report provided to ICU nurse, pt's family notified by MD ————————— Jane Klass, RN

> Events are documented in correct time sequence.

bracket around it, and write *See progress notes*. Then record the information fully and legibly in the notes.

No pencils, please

Because it's a permanent document, the clinical record should be completed in ink or by computer. Use only black or blue ink. Red and green ink — which are traditionally used on evening and night shifts — don't photocopy clearly. Also, don't use felt-tipped pens on forms with carbon copies because the pens usually don't hold up under the pressure needed to produce copies and the ink is more likely to bleed through to another page or smear if the paper gets wet.

Spelling counts

Notes filled with misspelled words and incorrect grammar create the same negative impression as illegible handwriting. Try hard to avoid these errors because information can be misrepresented or misconstrued if a medical record ends up in court. (*Tips for improving spelling and grammar,* page 194.)

Art of the chart

Neatness counts!

Make sure your handwriting is as neat and clear as possible. Legible charting is vital in communications between colleagues. The flowsheet below shows legible and illegible charting.

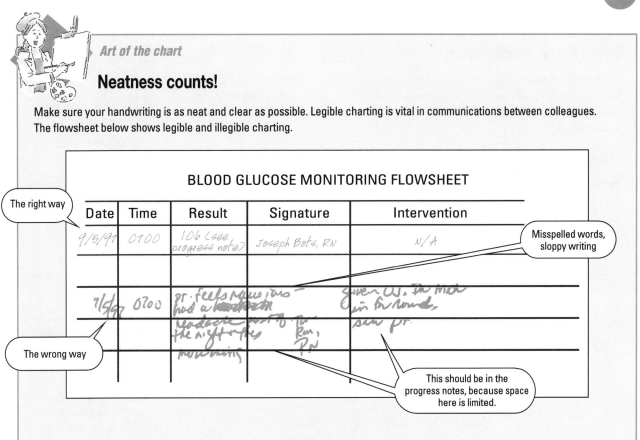

BLOOD GLUCOSE MONITORING FLOWSHEET

The right way

Date	Time	Result	Signature	Intervention
9/5/97	0100	106 (see progress note)	Joseph Bots, RN	N/A

The wrong way

Misspelled words, sloppy writing

This should be in the progress notes, because space here is limited.

Using abbreviations appropriately

Standards set by the Joint Commission on Accreditation of Healthcare Organizations (JCAHO) and many state regulations stipulate that health care facilities develop a list of approved abbreviations to use during charting. (See *Avoid these abbreviations!* pages 194 and 195.) Be sure that you know and use your facility's approved abbreviations. When you have doubts about an abbreviation's meaning, spell it out.

Using unapproved or ambiguous abbreviations can endanger a patient. For example, if you use *o.d.* for "once a day," another nurse might think you mean "oculus dexter" (right eye) and instill medication into the patient's eye instead of giving it orally. (See *Acceptable vs. unacceptable abbreviations*, page 196.)

Avoid these abbreviations!

The Joint Commission on Accreditation of Healthcare Organizations requires every health care facility to develop a list of approved abbreviations for staff use. Certain abbreviations should be avoided because they're easily misunderstood, especially when handwritten. Here's a list of those to avoid.

ABBREVIATION	INTENDED MEANING	CORRECTION
Apothecaries' symbols		
℥	fluid ounce	Use the metric equivalents
ʒ	fluid dram	Use the metric equivalents
♏	minim	Use the metric equivalents
℈	scruple	Use the metric equivalents
Drug names		
MTX	methotrexate	Use the complete spelling for drug names
CPZ	Compazine (prochlorperazine)	Use the complete spelling for drug names
HCl	hydrochloric acid	Use the complete spelling for drug names
DIG	digoxin	Use the complete spelling for drug names
MVI	multivitamins *without* fat-soluble vitamins	Use the complete spelling for drug names
HCTZ	hydrochlorothiazide	Use the complete spelling for drug names
ara-a	vidarabine	Use the complete spelling for drug names

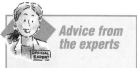
Tips for improving spelling and grammar

Want to look smart when you chart? Here are a few pointers:

☑ Keep both standard and medical dictionaries in charting areas and refer to them as needed.

☑ Post a list of commonly misspelled or confusing words, especially terms and medications regularly used on the unit. Many medications have very similar names but extremely different actions.

☑ If your computer system includes a spelling or grammar check, use it. Understand, though, that these are far from foolproof and don't take the place of careful proofreading.

Avoid these abbreviations! *(continued)*

ABBREVIATION	INTENDED MEANING	CORRECTION
Dosage directions		
aU	each ear	Write it out.
Mg	microgram	Use "mcg."
OD	once daily	Write it out. Don't abbreviate "daily."
OJ	orange juice	Write it out.
TID	once daily	Write it out.
Per os	orally	Use "P.O.," "by mouth," or "orally."
qn	nightly or at bedtime	Use "h.s." or "nightly."
subq	subcutaneous	Use "S.C." or write it out
U or U	unit	Write it out.

Correcting errors properly

When you make a mistake on a chart, correct it immediately by drawing a single line through the entry and writing *mistaken entry* above or beside it. Never erase a mistake, cover it with correction fluid, or completely cross it out, because this looks as if you're trying to hide something. Also, writing *oops* or *sorry,* or drawing a happy or sad face anywhere on a document is unprofessional and inappropriate. (See *Correct correctly!* page 197.)

Changing a record in any way is illegal and constitutes tampering. If the chart ends up in court, the plaintiff's lawyer will be looking for red flags that cast doubt on the chart's accuracy. So heed the following list of five don'ts:

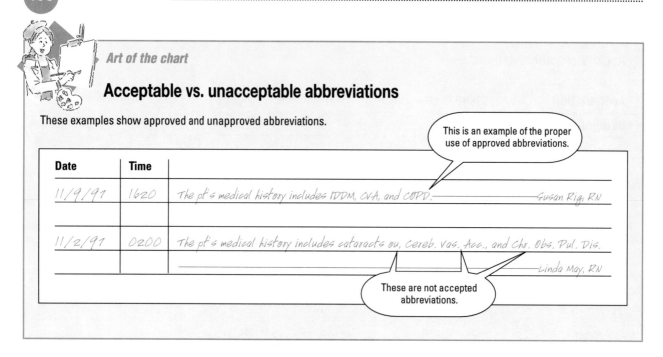

Art of the chart

Acceptable vs. unacceptable abbreviations

These examples show approved and unapproved abbreviations.

> This is an example of the proper use of approved abbreviations.

Date	Time	
11/9/91	1620	The pt's medical history includes IDDM, CVA, and COPD. ——————— Susan Rig, RN
11/2/91	0200	The pt's medical history includes cataracts ou, Cereb. Vas. Acc., and Chr. Obs. Pul. Dis. ——————— Linda May, RN

> These are not accepted abbreviations.

• Don't add information at a later date without indicating that you did so.
• Don't date the entry so it appears to have been written at an earlier time.
• Don't add inaccurate information.
• Don't omit information.
• Don't destroy records.

> An important charting rule: Never erase a mistake.

Signing documents

Sign each entry you make in your progress notes with your first name or initial, last name, and professional licensure (such as RN or LPN). Your employer may also require that you include your job title. If you find the last entry unsigned, immediately contact the nurse who made the entry and have her sign her name. If you can't locate her, simply write and sign your progress notes. The difference in charting times and handwriting should make it clear who the author was. (See *Charting do's and don'ts,* page 198.)

To be continued . . .

When charting continues from one page to the next, sign the bottom of the first page. At the top of

Art of the chart

Correct correctly!

When you make a mistake on the clinical record, correct it by drawing a single line through the entry and writing the words *mistaken entry* above or beside it (don't use an abbreviation like *m.e.*, which could be someone's initials). Follow this with your initials and the date. If appropriate, briefly explain why the correction was necessary.

Be sure that the mistaken entry is still readable. This indicates that you're only trying to correct a mistake, not cover something up.

Date	Time	Sign entries
11/10/91	0900	*Mistaken entry N.C. 11/10/91* ~~Pt. states he is dizzy when changing from sitting to standing position~~
		————————————————————— *Nancy Cobb, RN*

> The right way to correct an error

> The wrong, legally improper way

---

the next page, write the date, time, and *continued from previous page.* Be sure each page is stamped or labeled with the patient's identifying information.

Never leave blank spaces on forms. This implies that you failed to give complete care or to assess the patient completely. If information listed on a form doesn't apply to your patient, write *N/A* (not applicable) in the space. If your charting doesn't fill the designated space, draw a line through the empty space until you reach your signature.

What you didn't see can hurt you

If you need to chart the actions of nursing assistants or technicians, write the caregiver's full name, not just his initials. Many nurses worry about countersigning care that they didn't actually see performed. If you feel this way, you may refer to your facility's policy, contact your state board of nursing, or discuss the issue with your nurse manager. *Remember, your signature makes you responsible for everything in the notes.*

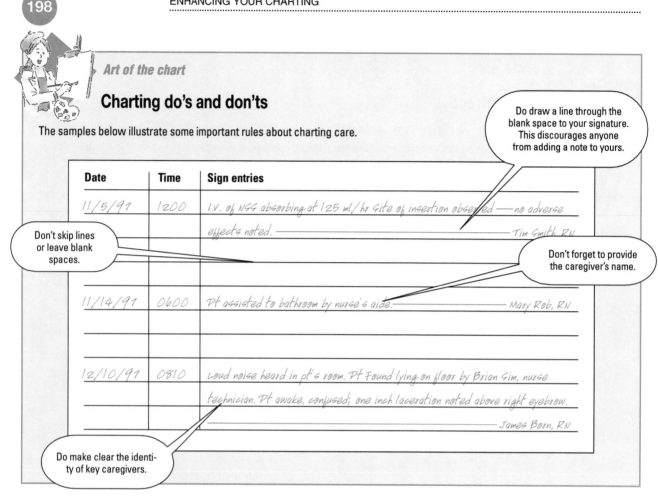

Art of the chart

Charting do's and don'ts

The samples below illustrate some important rules about charting care.

Do draw a line through the blank space to your signature. This discourages anyone from adding a note to yours.

Date	Time	Sign entries
11/5/91	1200	I.V. of NSS absorbing at 125 ml/hr Site of insertion observed —no adverse effects noted. ————————————— Tim Smith, RN
11/14/91	0600	Pt assisted to bathroom by nurse's aide.———————— Mary Rob, RN
12/10/91	0810	Loud noise heard in pt's room. Pt found lying on floor by Brian Sim, nurse technician. Pt awake, confused; one inch laceration noted above right eyebrow. ————————————— James Born, RN

Don't skip lines or leave blank spaces.

Don't forget to provide the caregiver's name.

Do make clear the identity of key caregivers.

Doctors' orders

Almost every treatment you give a patient requires a doctor's order, so accurate documentation of these orders is critical. Doctors' orders fall into four categories:
- written orders
- preprinted orders
- verbal orders
- telephone orders.

Written orders

No matter who transcribes a doctor's order — an RN, LPN, or unit secretary — a second person must double-check the transcription for accuracy. An effective method used by many facilities is the "chart check" — rechecking orders from the previous shift once per shift.

Checking for transcription errors at least once every 24 hours is also a good idea. These checks are usually done on the night shift. A line is placed across the order sheet to indicate that all orders above the line have been checked. Then the sheet is signed and dated to verify that the check was done.

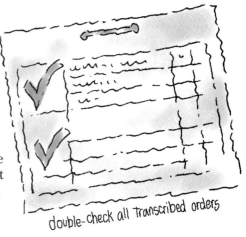

double-check all transcribed orders

Heading off mistakes

When checking a patient's order sheet, make sure that the orders were written for the right patient. An order sheet might be stamped with one patient's identification plate and then inadvertently placed in another patient's chart. Double-checking averts potential mistakes.

If an order is unclear, call the doctor who wrote the order for clarification. Don't ask other people for their interpretation; they'll only be guessing, too. If a doctor is notorious for his poor handwriting, ask him to read his orders to you before he leaves the unit.

Preprinted orders

Many health care facilities use preprinted order forms to make doctors' orders easier to read and interpret. Such forms are especially useful for commonly performed procedures such as cardiac catheterization. As with other standardized documents, blanks are used for information that must be individualized according to the patient's needs.

If your facility uses these forms, don't assume that they're flawless just because they're preprinted. You may still need to clarify an order by discussing it with the doctor who gave it. (See *Preprinted orders,* page 200.)

Verbal orders

Verbal orders are easy to misinterpret. Errors in understanding or documenting such orders can cause mistakes

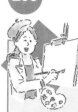

Art of the chart

Preprinted orders

The following is an example of a preprinted form for charting doctors' orders. This form specifies the treatment for a patient who is about to undergo cardiac catheterization.

DOCTOR'S ORDERS

Allergies: *None known*

Date/Time	PRECARDIAC CATHETERIZATION ORDERS:
12/1/91 0130	1. NPO after _midnight_ except for medications.
	2. Shave and prep right and left groin areas.
	3. Premedications:
	Benadryl _25_ mg
	Xanax _0.5_ mg } P.O. on call to Cath lab
	4. Have ECG, PT, PTT, Creatinine, Hgb, Hct, and platelet count
	on chart prior to sending the patient to the Cath lab.
	5. Have patient void before leaving for the Cath lab.
12/1/91 0200	*Mona Jones, RN*

> Blanks are left for information that should be individualized according to the patient's needs.

---

in patient care and liability problems for you and your facility. So try to take verbal orders only in an emergency when the doctor can't immediately attend to the patient. As a rule, do-not-resuscitate and no-code orders should *not* be taken verbally.

From words to paper

Carefully follow your facility's policy for documenting verbal orders, using a special form if one exists. Here's the usual procedure:

• Record the order on the doctor's order sheet as soon as possible. Note the date and time.
• On the first line, write *V.O.* for verbal order. Then write the doctor's name and your name as the nurse who received and read the order back to the doctor.
• Record the order verbatim.
• Sign your name.
• Draw lines through any space between the order and your verification of the order.
• Write in ink the type of drug, the dosage, the time you administered it, and any other information. (See *Charting verbal orders*.)

Make sure that the doctor countersigns the order within the time limits set by your facility. Without his countersignature, you may be held liable for practicing medicine without a license.

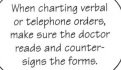

When charting verbal or telephone orders, make sure the doctor reads and counter-signs the forms.

Telephone orders

Ideally, you should accept only written orders from a doctor. But telephone orders are permissible in the following circumstances:
• The patient needs immediate treatment and the doctor isn't available to write an order.

▶ *Art of the chart*

Charting verbal orders

This form shows the correct way to chart verbal orders.

Date/time	Sign entries
11/16/91 1500	V.O. Dr. Marks to Mary Jones, RN
	Lasix 40 mg-I.V. now and daily starting in a.m.
	Mary Jones, RN

• You are providing care to the patient at home. If so, the orders must be signed by the doctor according to state nursing practice regulations. Under Medicare guidelines, verbal orders must be signed within 30 days. Other agencies impose their own, stricter rules. Failure to obtain a signed order could jeopardize reimbursement.

• New information (laboratory data, for example) has become available and the telephone order will enable you to expedite care. (See *Taking telephone orders*.)

From phone to paper

Telephone orders should be given directly to you; they should never go through a third party. Carefully follow your facility's policy for documenting these orders. Usually, you'll follow this procedure:

• Record the order on the doctor's order sheet as soon as possible. First, note the date and time. On the next line, write *T.O.* for telephone order. (Don't use "P.O." for phone order; it could be mistaken for "by mouth.") Then write the doctor's name and sign your name.

• Write the order verbatim.

• If you're having trouble understanding the doctor, ask another nurse to listen in as the doctor gives you the order. Then have her sign the order, too.

• Draw lines through any blank spaces in the order.

• Make sure that the doctor countersigns the order within the time limits set by your facility. Without his signature,

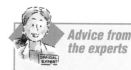

Advice from the experts

When in doubt, check it out

An order may be correct when issued, but incorrect later because of changes in the patient's status. When this occurs, delay the treatment until you've contacted the doctor and clarified the situation.

Failure to question

In *Poor Sisters of Saint Francis Seraph of the Perpetual Adoration, et al. v. Catron (1982),* a hospital was sued for negligence because a nurse failed to question a doctor's order regarding an endotracheal tube.

The doctor ordered that the tube be left in place for 5 days instead of the standard 2 to 3 days. The nurse knew that 5 days was exceptionally long, but instead of clarifying the doctor's order and documenting her actions, she followed the order. As a result, the patient's larynx was irreparably damaged, and the court ruled the hospital negligent.

Art of the chart

Taking telephone orders

This form shows the correct way to chart telephone orders.

Date/Time	Sign entries
12/4/91 0900	T.O. Dr. Bartholomew White to Cathy Phillips, RN
	Demerol 75 mg and Vistaril 50 mg I.M. now for pain.
	—— Cathy Phillips, RN

you may be held liable for practicing medicine without a license.

• To save time and avoid errors (and if permitted by your facility's confidentiality policy), ask the doctor to fax you a copy of the order. Make sure you wait at the fax machine for the transmission, to protect the patient's right to confidentiality.

Questioning doctors' orders

Although the unit secretary may transcribe orders, you're ultimately responsible for the transcription's accuracy. Only you have the authority and the knowledge to question the validity of orders and to spot errors.

Stop, question, and chart

What if an order seems vague or even wrong? Refuse to carry it out until you talk to the doctor. (See *When in doubt, check it out*.) Your facility should have a written procedure for clarifying orders. If it doesn't, take these steps:

• Contact the prescribing doctor for clarification.
• Document that you did this.
• Document whether you carried out the order.
• If you refuse to carry out an order, document your refusal, including the reasons why you refused and your communications with the doctor. Inform your immediate supervisor.
• Ask your nursing administrator for a step-by-step policy to follow so you'll know what to do if the situation recurs.

Sometimes, an order is correct when it's given, then becomes incorrect later because the patient's status changes. When this occurs, delay the treatment until you've contacted the doctor for clarification.

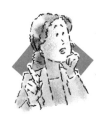

Quick quiz

1. When documenting objectively, you should chart:
   A. what you see, hear, and do.
   B. the opinions of the health care team.
   C. what you think the patient's response will be.

Answer: A. Objective statements include facts, not opinions or assumptions.

2. When documenting events in a patient's chart, you should:
   A. chart the period of time the shift covers, such as 0700 to 1500 hours.
   B. chart the specific time of each event.
   C. chart every hour on the hour.

Answer: B. Chart the exact time of all sudden changes in a patient's condition, significant events, and nursing actions.

3. Assessments and observations should be charted in chronological order because:
   A. they'll reveal a pattern of improvement or deterioration.
   B. it's more convenient to chart this way.
   C. the JCAHO requires it.

Answer: A. Usually, an isolated assessment tells us very little about a patient.

Scoring

☆☆　If you answered all three items correctly, wow! Your charting is complete, concise, accurate, etc. Turn to the next chapter and keep mastering the art of the chart.

☆　If you answered fewer than three correctly, don't worry! In keeping with the tenets of good charting, we'll keep it confidential.

Avoiding legal pitfalls

Just the facts

In this chapter you'll learn:

♦ the legal significance of the medical record

♦ how to chart defensively

♦ the relationship between charting and risk management

♦ eight charting pitfalls.

A look at legal pitfalls in charting

As your professional responsibility grows, so does your legal accountability. Complete, accurate documentation proves that you're giving quality care and meeting the standards set by the nursing profession, your health care facility, and the law. It's your best protection if you're named in a malpractice lawsuit. (See *What sways the jury?* page 206.)

Communication is primary

Although faulty charting is a pivotal issue in many malpractice cases, only a tiny number of medical records actually end up in court. If you think of the medical record as a communication tool and document accordingly, you won't panic if the court subpoenas it. But if you focus on the legal implications and document just to protect yourself, your charting will sound self-serving, defensive, and one-sided to the judge and jury.

> Remember, charts are communication tools first and foremost.

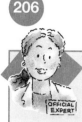

What sways the jury?

The outcome of every malpractice trial boils down to one question: Whom will the jury believe? The answer depends on the credibility of the evidence. Jurors usually view the medical record as the best evidence of what really happened. It's often the hinge on which the verdict swings.

A general overview

In a nutshell, here's what happens in court: The plaintiff's (patient's) lawyer presents evidence showing that the patient was harmed because care provided by the defendant (in this case, the nurse) failed to meet accepted standards. The nurse's lawyer presents evidence showing that his client provided an acceptable standard of care.

   If the nurse wasn't negligent, the medical record is her best friend because it provides evidence of quality care. But if she *was* negligent and truthfully documented her care, the medical record is the plaintiff's best evidence. The jury will almost certainly rule in favor of the patient.

Legal standards

What and how you chart on the medical record is controlled by:
- nurse practice acts
- American Nurses Association (ANA) standards
- malpractice litigation
- your facility's policies and procedures.

Nurse practice acts

Nurse practice acts are state laws that designate what a nurse can do in that state. Today, nurses are considered managers of care as well as practitioners; states revise their laws and documentation requirements to keep up with changes like this in the nursing profession.

ANA standards

What you write in a medical record shouldn't be dictated by the courts; it should be controlled by the nursing profession's own standards. Charting that meets these standards describes the patient's status, medical treatment, and nursing care. The ANA sets standards for most nursing specialties. It says that documentation must be:
- systematic

- continuous
- accessible
- communicated
- recorded
- readily available to all members of the health care team.

Go with the flow sheet

Documentation goals haven't changed much over the years, but documentation methods have. Nurses now use flow sheets, graphic records, and checklists in place of long narrative notes. In malpractice cases, the charting method used isn't important, as long as it's used consistently and provides comprehensive, factual information that's relevant to the patient's care.

Malpractice litigation

When charting, your main goal is to convey information. But keep the legal implications in the back of your mind. If the care you provide and your charting are both top-notch, the records may be used to refute a plaintiff's accusation of nursing malpractice.

A malpractice verdict depends on these three factors:
- breach of duty
- damage
- causation.

A relationship means responsibility

The courts have ruled that your duty is to provide an appropriate standard of care once a nurse-patient relationship is established — even if the relationship takes place over the phone. Breach of duty means that your care didn't meet that standard.

Proving that a nurse was guilty of breach of duty is difficult because her duties overlap with those of other health care providers. The court will ask: "How would a reasonable, prudent nurse with comparable training and experience have acted in the same or a similar circumstance?"

Once the plaintiff establishes a breach of duty, he must then prove that the breach caused the patient's injury (damage and causation).

> Once you establish a relationship with a patient, you take on a legal responsibility.

Facility policies and procedures

How you chart is also controlled by the policies and procedures in your facility's employee and nursing manuals. Straying from these rules suggests that you failed to meet the facility's standards of care.

Although the courts haven't decided whether these policies actually establish a standard of care, in every nursing malpractice case the nurse's actions are compared with the appropriate standard of care. The courts use regularly updated, national minimum standards established by professional organizations and accrediting bodies as guidelines.

> Establishing a strong nurse-patient relationship may help reduce legal risks.

The long arm of the law

According to insurance company data, lawsuits naming nurses as defendants are increasing. Why? Nurses' expanding roles and the breakdown of the nurse-patient relationship due to shorter hospital stays are two reasons. Developing a rapport with your patients, even on a short-term basis, can help decrease errors and foster a nurse-patient relationship; both of which help prevent lawsuits.

Charting defensively

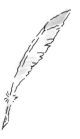

As they say in the sports world, "The best offense is a good defense." In the world of nursing and malpractice, the best way to avoid having to defend yourself in court is to chart factually and defensively. This involves knowing:
- how to chart
- what to chart
- when to chart
- who should chart.

How to chart

A skilled nurse charts with a jury in mind and knows that how she charts is just as important as what she charts.

Rule #1: Stick to the facts

Record only what you see, hear, smell, feel, measure, and count, not what you suppose, infer, conclude, or assume. For example, if a patient pulled out his I.V. line, but you didn't witness it, write: *Found pt, arm board, and bed linens covered with blood. I.V. line and venipuncture device were untaped and hanging free.* If the patient says he pulled out his I.V. line, record that.

Don't chart your opinions. If the chart is used as evidence in court, the plaintiff's lawyer might attack your credibility and the medical record's reliability. You can chart subjective information, but only when it's supported by documented facts.

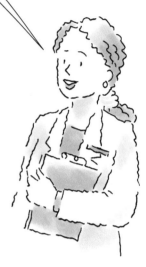

Remember, facts speak for themselves. Never chart subjective information unless you have solid facts to back it up.

Rule #2: Avoid labeling

Objectively describe the patient's behavior instead of subjectively labeling it. Expressions like *appears spaced out, flying high, exhibiting bizarre behavior,* or *using obscenities* mean different things to different people. Could you define these terms in court? Objectivity in charting may increase your credibility with the jury.

Rule #3: Be specific

Your charting goal is to present the facts clearly and concisely. To do so, use only approved abbreviations and express your observations in quantifiable terms.(See *Specifics are terrific!*)

For example, writing *output adequate* isn't as helpful as writing *output 1,200 ml.* And *Pt appears to be in pain* is vague compared to *Pt requested pain medication after complaining of severe lower back pain radiating to his right leg.*

Art of the chart

Specifics are terrific!

The note below is clear and concise because it uses approved abbreviations and specific measurements.

10/16/91	1100	Complaining of pain at left antecubital I.V. site at 1000. Dressing removed.
		Redness 2 cm wide around insertion site. No drainage. Quarter-sized area of
		edema above insertion site. I.V. removed; site cleaned with povidone-iodine
		and sterile dressing applied. Warm compress applied to site X 20 min.
		Acetaminophen 650 mg given P.O. at 1015. Pt reports relief.————————
		———————————————————— Margaret Doherty, RN

Also avoid catch-all phrases like *Pt comfortable.* Instead, describe how you know this. For instance, is the patient resting, reading, or sleeping?

Rule #4: Use neutral language

Don't use inappropriate comments or language in your notes. This is unprofessional and can cause legal problems.

In one case, an elderly patient developed pressure ulcers, and his family complained that he wasn't receiving adequate care. The patient later died, probably of natural causes. Because family members were dissatisfied with the patient's care, they sued. The insurance company questioned the abbreviation *PBBB* in the chart, which the doctor had written under prognosis. After learning that this stood for "pine box by bedside," the family was awarded a significant sum.

Rule #5: Eliminate bias

Don't use language that suggests a negative attitude toward the patient. Examples include *obstinate, drunk, obnoxious, bizarre,* or *abusive.* The same goes for what you say out loud and then document. Disparaging remarks, accusations, arguments, or name calling could lead to a defamation of character or libel suit. In court, the plaintiff's lawyer might say, "This nurse called my client 'rude, difficult, and uncooperative.' It's right here in her own handwriting! No wonder she didn't take good care of him — she didn't like him." *Remember, the patient has a legal right to see his chart. If he spots a derogatory reference, he'll be hurt, angry, and more likely to sue.*

If a patient is difficult or uncooperative, document the behavior objectively and let the jurors draw their own conclusions. (See *Polite and to the point.*)

Rule # 6: Keep the record intact

Be sure to keep the patient's chart complete. Discarding pages, even for innocent reasons, raises doubt in a lawyer's mind.

Let's say that you spill coffee on a page and blur several entries. Don't discard the original! Copy it and put the copy and the original in the chart. Then cross-reference the pages by writing, *Recopied from page___* on the copy and *Recopied on page___* on the original.

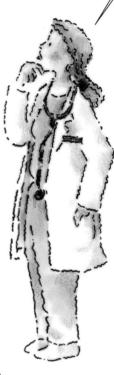

Inappropriate or flip comments in your chart increase your legal risks.

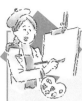

Art of the chart

Polite and to the point

The note below describes a difficult situation dispassionately, while still getting the point across.

11/17/91	1300	I attempted to perform the daily abdominal dressing change, but pt stated, "This doesn't need to be done every day. It doesn't hurt and I don't want you to touch it. Leave me alone." I explained the importance of monitoring and cleaning the incision, and offered an analgesic to be given 20 minutes before dressing would be changed. Pt became agitated and still refused. Dr. Humbert notified that incisional site was not assessed nor was dressing changed, and that patient is agitated. ———————— Mary Marley, RN

What to chart

Caring for patients seems more important than documenting every detail, doesn't it? But legally speaking, an incomplete chart reflects incomplete nursing care. Deleting details is such a serious and common charting error that malpractice lawyers have coined the expression "Not charted, not done."

This doesn't mean that you have to document everything. Some information, like staffing shortages and staff conflicts, is definitely off limits. (See *Charting don'ts,* page 212.) But other information absolutely must be charted.

Rule #1: Chart significant situations

Learn to recognize legally dangerous situations as you give patient care. (See *A case of negligence,* page 213.) Assess each critical or out of the ordinary situation and decide whether your actions might be significant in court. If they could be, chart them, as well as every other detail of the situation. (See *Out of the ordinary,* page 214.)

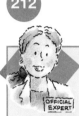

Advice from the experts

Charting don'ts

Negative language and inappropriate information don't belong in a medical record and can return to haunt you in a lawsuit. The charting mistakes below are legal land mines. Avoid them.

1. Don't record staffing problems.
True, staff shortages may affect patient care or contribute to an incident. But don't mention this in a patient's chart; it can be used as legal ammunition against you if the chart lands in court. Instead, write a confidential memo to your nurse-manager, and review your facility's policy and procedure manuals to see how you're expected to handle this situation.

2. Don't record staff conflicts.
Don't chart:
• disputes with other nurses (including criticisms of their care)
• questions about a doctor's treatment
• a colleague's rude or abusive behavior.
Personality clashes aren't legitimate patient care concerns. In the event of a lawsuit, the plaintiff's lawyer will exploit conflicts among codefendants.

   Instead of charting these problems, talk with your nurse-manager, or consult with the doctor directly if an order puzzles you. If another nurse writes personal accusations or charges of incompetence in a chart, talk to her about the implications of doing this.

3. Don't mention incident reports.
Incident reports are confidential and filed separately from the patient's chart. Document only the facts of an incident in the chart, and never write "incident report" or indicate that you filed one.

   For example, write: *Found pt lying on the floor at 1250 hours. Vital signs were stable. Notified Dr. Gary Dietrich at 1253 hours, and he saw pt at 1300 hours.*

4. Don't use words associated with errors.
Terms like "by mistake," "accidentally," "somehow," "unintentionally," "miscalculated," and "confusing" are bonus words to the plaintiff's attorney. Steer clear of words that suggest an error was made or a patient's safety was jeopardized. Let the facts speak for themselves.

   For example, suppose you gave a patient 100 mg of Demerol instead of 50 mg. Here's how to chart this without calling undue attention to it: *Pt was given Demerol 100 mg I.M. at 1300 hours for abdominal pain. Dr. was notified but gave no orders. Pt's vital signs remained stable.*

5. Don't name a second patient.
Naming a second patient in a patient's chart violates confidentiality. Instead, write *roommate,* the patient's initials, or his room and bed number.

6. Don't chart casual conversations with colleagues.
Telling your nurse-manager in the elevator or restroom about a patient's deteriorating condition doesn't qualify as informing her. She's likely to forget the details, or may not even realize you expect her to intervene. Before notifying someone, clearly state why you're notifying the person so she can focus on the facts and take appropriate action. Otherwise, you can't chart that you informed her.

A case of negligence

Here's a fictional case that exemplifies how negligence may be interpreted in court.

Seventeen-year old Tommy York was partially paralyzed and severely brain damaged after an accident. He was admitted to the hospital for an intensive rehabilitation program.

Soon afterward, his parents told the nurse that a support from the right side of his wheelchair was missing and that they saw scratches on his right arm. Although the nurse also noticed this, she didn't record it.

Failure to document

Later, the patient's hip became red, swollen, and increasingly painful. His mother also reported these symptoms to the nurse, who again failed to record them in the medical record.

When the patient was finally diagnosed with a broken hip, his parents sued. The court ruled the hospital negligent and awarded the plaintiff $250,000.

A matter of duty

Inadequate observation of patients that leads to misdiagnosis or injury is a common cause of lawsuits involving nurses. Most of these lawsuits involve issues of negligence — the failure to exercise the degree of care that a person of ordinary prudence would exercise under the same circumstances. A claim of negligence requires that there be a duty owed by one person to another, that the duty be breached, and that injury result.

Malpractice is a more restricted, specialized type of negligence, defined as a violation of professional duty to act with reasonable care and in good faith. Several states have begun to recognize nursing negligence as a form of malpractice.

Avoid negligence cases by documenting any and all unusual patient events.

Rule #2: Chart complete assessment data

Failing to perform and document a complete physical assessment is a key factor in many malpractice suits. During your initial assessment, focus on the patient's chief complaint, and then follow up on all other problems he mentions. Be sure to chart everything you do and why.

After completing the initial assessment, write a well-constructed plan of care. This gives you a clear approach to the patient's problems and helps defend your care if you're sued.

Phrase each problem statement clearly, and modify them as you gather new assessment data. State the plan of care for solving each problem; then identify the actions you intend to take.

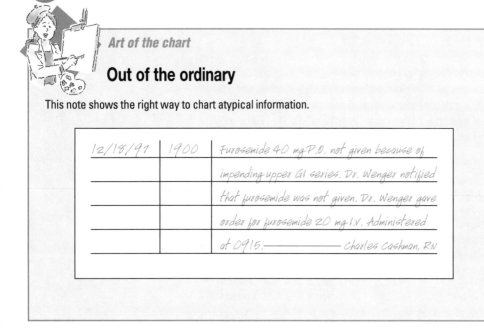

Art of the chart

Out of the ordinary

This note shows the right way to chart atypical information.

12/18/91	1900	Furosemide 40 mg P.O. not given because of impending upper GI series. Dr. Wenger notified that furosemide was not given. Dr. Wenger gave order for furosemide 20 mg I.V. Administered at 0915.————————— Charles Cashman, RN

Rule #3: Document discharge instructions

Because of insurance constraints, facilities are discharging patients earlier than they used to. This means that patients and family members are changing dressings, assessing wounds, and tackling other tasks that nurses traditionally performed.

Patient and family teaching is usually your responsibility. If a patient receives inadequate or incorrect instructions and an injury results, you could be held liable.

Many facilities give patients printed instruction sheets that describe treatments and home care procedures. In court, these materials may be used as evidence that instruction took place. To support testimony, they should be tailored to each patient's specific needs and contain any verbal or written instructions you provided. Documentation of referrals to home health care agencies or other community providers is another essential component of discharge planning.

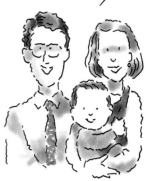

Teaching us is part of your professional responsibility.

When to chart

Finding time to chart can be hard during a busy shift. But the timeliness of entries is a major issue in malpractice suits.

Rule #1

Document nursing care when you perform it or shortly afterward. Never document ahead of time — your notes will be inaccurate and you'll leave out information about the patient's response to treatment. Even if you did what you charted, a lawyer might ask "Do you occasionally chart something before doing it?" If you answer yes, the jury won't see the chart as a reliable indicator of what you actually did, which wrecks your credibility.

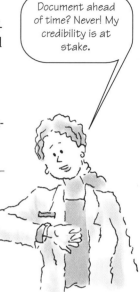

Document ahead of time? Never! My credibility is at stake.

Who should chart

State nurse practice acts have strict rules about who can chart. Breaking these rules can cause you to have your nursing license suspended.

Rule # 1

No matter how busy you are, never ask another nurse to complete your charting (and never complete another nurse's charting). Doing so is a dangerous practice that may be specifically prohibited by your state's nurse practice act. If the other nurse makes an error or misinterprets information, the patient can be harmed. Then, if he sues you for negligence, both you and your facility will be held accountable because delegated documentation doesn't meet nursing standards.

Delegating charting has another consequence: It destroys the credibility and value of the medical record both in the facility and in court. Judges give little if any weight to medical records containing secondhand observations or hearsay evidence.

Risk management and documentation

A health care facility's reputation for safe, reliable, effective service is its main defense against liability claims. Well-coordinated risk management and quality improvement programs show the public that the facility is being managed in a legally responsible manner. If complaints arise, a good program ensures that they're handled promptly to contain the damage and minimize liability claims. (See *Understanding risk management and quality improvement*, page 216.)

Records reveal potential risk

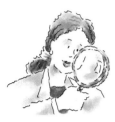

Sometimes documentation reveals potential problems within a health care facility. For example, a certain procedure may repeatedly lead to patient injury or another type of accident. Risk management programs help reduce injuries and accidents and thereby minimize financial loss.

In the past, the focus of risk management and quality improvement programs was to maintain and improve facilities and equipment and ensure employee, visitor, and patient safety. But today, the focus is on identifying, evaluating, and reducing patient injury in specialty units that have the greatest malpractice risks.

Preventing adverse events

Risk management has three main goals:

☞ decreasing the number of claims by promptly identifying and following up on adverse events (early warning systems)

☞ reducing the frequency of preventable injuries and accidents leading to lawsuits by maintaining or improving the quality of care

☞ controlling costs related to claims by pinpointing trouble spots early and working with the patient and his family.

Early warning systems

Early warning systems can pinpoint much useful information, but to be effective they need:
• a strong organizational structure
• cooperation between risk management and quality improvement departments
• the commitment of all staff members to report adverse events to the appropriate clinical chairperson, so he can study the medical records more closely or talk to the staff member involved and recommend remedial education, monitoring, or restricted privileges
• the commitment of key staff members — such as nurses, doctors, administrators, and chiefs of high-risk services — to analyze the information.

The most commonly used early warning systems are occurrence reporting and occurrence screening.

Understanding risk management and quality improvement

Do the terms *risk management* and *quality improvement* confuse you? Here's how to tell them apart: Risk management focuses on patients' and family members' perceptions of the care provided, whereas quality improvement focuses on the role of the health care provider.

Many facilities combine these two programs in their educational efforts. They place a high priority on teaching new medical residents and nurses about malpractice claims, staff members' reporting obligations, proper informational and reporting channels, and principles of risk management and quality improvement.

Occurrence reporting

An occurrence or incident report refers to the documentation of events that are inconsistent with a health care facility's ordinary routine, regardless of whether injury occurs. Doctors, nurses, or other staff are responsible for reporting such events when they are observed or shortly afterward. Examples include the unplanned return of a patient to the operating room or a medication error.

Occurrence screening

Occurrence screening involves reviewing medical records to find adverse events. Both general indicators of adverse events, such as a nosocomial infection or medication error, and more specific indicators, such as an incorrect sponge count during surgery, are considered.

Occurrence screening requires careful review of medical records.

Managing incidents

Despite risk management programs, adverse events still occur. Health care facilities rely on the following sources to identify dangerous situations or trends:

• *Incident reports.* Also called occurrence reports, incident reports are a primary source of information for lawyers, too. They use the reports when researching potential lawsuits and in court as evidence.

• *Nurses.* Nurses are usually the first ones to recognize potential problems because they spend so much time with patients and families. They know which patients are dissatisfied with their care and which ones have complications that may lead to injuries.

• *Patient-representative office.* Patient representatives keep files of patient complaints, identify litigious patients, and maintain contact with the patient and his family after an incident has occurred.

• *Business office and medical records department.* People in these offices may be alerted to potential lawsuits when a patient threatens to sue after he receives his bill or when a patient or a lawyer requests a copy of the medical record.

• *Other sources.* The engineering department has information on the safety of the hospital environment. Purchasing, biomedical engineering, and the pharmacy can report on the safety and adequacy of products and equipment. Social workers, hospital clergy, volunteers, and patient escorts often know about highly dissatisfied patients.

Remember: Whenever you get a report from one of these sources, document it thoroughly on the patient's medical record and fill out an incident report.

Claim notice chain reaction

Once the risk manager learns of a potential or actual lawsuit, he notifies the medical records department and the facility's insurance company. The medical records department makes copies of the patient's chart and files the original in a safe place to prevent tampering.

A claim notice should also trigger a quality improvement peer review of the medical record. This review measures the health care provider's conduct against the professional standards of conduct for the particular situation. This information is used by the risk manager to investigate the claim's merit and the facility's responsibility in that situation. The standard required for a successful defense isn't always as high as the facility's optimal standard.

Following the guidelines here will reduce your legal risks.

Eight legal hazards

Every day, you face patient care situations that could land you in court. Your challenge is to watch out for these occurrences and chart them defensively without becoming obsessive about it. The section that follows describes eight volatile legal situations.

Hazard #1: Incident reports

Whenever you witness an adverse event, file an incident report. (See *Completing an incident report.*) Some things to report are injuries from restraints, burns, or other causes; falls (even if the patient wasn't injured); and a patient's insistence on being discharged against medical advice. If an incident report form doesn't leave enough space to fully describe an incident, attach an additional page of comments.

The form's function

An incident report isn't part of the patient's chart, but it may be used later in litigation. A report has two functions:

Art of the chart

Completing an incident report

When you witness a reportable event, you must fill out an incident report. Forms vary, but most include the following information.

INCIDENT REPORT

Name _Greta Manning_
Address _1 Worth Way, Boston, MA_
Phone _(617) 555-1122_

| 9. DATE OF INCIDENT | 10. TIME OF INCIDENT |
| 11-14-91 | 1442 |

Addressograph if patient

11. EXACT LOCATION OF INCIDENT (Bldg., Floor, Room No., Area)
4-Main, Rm. 441

12. TYPE OF INCIDENT (CHECK ONE ONLY) □ PATIENT □ EMPLOYEE ☑ VISITOR □ VOLUNTEER □ OTHER (Specify)

13. DESCRIPTION OF THE INCIDENT (WHO, WHAT, WHEN, WHERE, HOW, WHY) (Use Back of Form if Necessary)

Wife of pt found on floor next to bed. States she was trying to put siderail of bed down to sit on pt's bed and fell down.

Describe relevant conditions.

State only what you saw or heard.

PATIENT FALL INCIDENTS

14. FLOOR CONDITIONS □ OTHER _____ ☑ CLEAN & SMOOTH □ SLIPPERY (WET)
FRAME OF BED ☑ LOW □ HIGH
NIGHT LIGHT □ YES ☑ NO

15. WERE BED RAILS PRESENT? □ NO □ 1 UP □ 2 UP □ 3 UP ☑ 4 UP
17. OTHER RESTRAINTS (TYPE & EXTENT) _N/A_

18. AMBULATION PRIVILEGE □ UNLIMITED □ LIMITED WITH ASSISTANCE □ COMPLETE BEDREST □ OTHER

19. WAS NARCOTICS, ANALGESICS, HYPNOTICS, SEDATIVES, DIURETICS, ANTIHYPERTENSIVES OR ANTICONVULSANTS GIVEN DURING LAST 4 HOURS? □ YES ☑ NO
DRUG AMOUNT TIME

PATIENT INCIDENTS

20. PHYSICIAN NOTIFIED NAME OF PHYSICIAN _J. Reynolds, MD_ DATE _11-14-91_ TIME _1445_ COMPLETE IF APPLICABLE

EMPLOYEE INCIDENTS

21. DEPARTMENT | 22. JOB TITLE | 23. SOCIAL SECURITY #
24. MARITAL STATUS

ALL INCIDENTS

27. SUPERVISOR NOTIFIED NAME OF SUPERVISOR _C. Jones, RN_ DATE _11-14-91_ TIME _1500_ | 28. LOCATION (WHERE TREATMENT WAS RENDERED)

29. NAME, ADDRESS AND TELEPHONE NUMBER OF WITNESS(ES) OR PERSONS FAMILIAR WITH INCIDENT - WITNESS OR NOT.
Connie Smith, RN (617)555-0912 1 Main St., Boston, MA

Names of those involved.

30. SIGNATURE OF PERSON PREPARING REPORT _Connie Smith_ | TITLE _RN_ | 31. DATE OF REPORT _11-14-91_

PHYSICIAN'S REPORT - To be completed for all cases involving injury or illness (DO NOT USE ABBREVIATIONS) (Use back of Form if necessary)

DIAGNOSIS AND TREATMENT
Received patient in Emergency Department after reported fall in husband's room. 12 cm x 12 cm ecchymotic area noted on right hip. X-rays negative for fracture. Good range of motion. Ice pack applied. ———— J. Reynolds, MD

33. DISPOSITION _sent home_

34. PERSON NOTIFIED OTHER THAN HOSPITAL PERSONNEL NAME AND ADDRESS _R. Manning (daughter) address same as pt_ | 35. DATE _11-14-91_ | 36. TIME _1500_

37. PHYSICIAN'S SIGNATURE _J. Reynolds, MD_ | 38. DATE _11-14-91_

☝ It informs the administration of the incident so the risk management staff can work on preventing similar incidents

✌ It alerts the administration and the facility's insurance company to a potential claim and the need for further investigation.

Eyewitness report

Only people who witnessed an incident should fill out and sign an incident report, and each witness should file a separate report. Once the report is filed, it may be reviewed by the nursing supervisor, the doctor who examined the patient after the incident, various department heads and administrators, the facility's attorney, and the insurance company.

Because incident reports will be read by many people and may even turn up in court, you must follow strict guidelines when completing them. (See *Tips for reporting incidents.*)

Revise and computerize

Facilities are continually revising their incident report forms; some have begun to use computerized forms. Incident reports are also processed by computer, which permits classifying and counting of incidents to indicate trends.

Charting incidents in progress notes

When documenting an incident in the medical record, follow these guidelines:

• Write a factual account of the incident, including treatment and follow-up care and the patient's response. This shows that the patient was closely monitored after the incident. Make sure the descriptions in the chart match those in the incident report.

> What I document in the incident report...

> ...has to match the information in the medical record.

Advice from the experts

Tips for reporting incidents

In the past, a plaintiff's lawyer wasn't allowed to see incident reports. Today, however, many states allow lawyers access to incident reports if they make their requests through proper channels. So, when writing an incident report, keep in mind who may read it and follow these guidelines:

Include essential information, such as the identity of the person involved in the incident, the exact time and place of the incident, and the name of the doctor you notified.

Document any unusual occurrences that you witnessed.

Record the events and the consequences for the patient in enough detail that administrators can decide whether or not to investigate further.

Write objectively, avoiding opinions, judgments, conclusions, or assumptions about who or what caused the incident. Tell your opinions to your supervisor or the risk manager later.

Describe only what you saw and heard and the actions you took to provide care at the scene. Unless you saw a patient fall, write *Found patient lying on the floor.*

Don't admit that you're at fault or blame someone else. Steer clear of statements like *Better staffing would have prevented this incident.*

Don't offer suggestions about how to prevent the incident from happening again.

Don't include detailed statements from witnesses and descriptions of remedial action; these are normally part of an investigative follow-up.

Don't put the report in the medical record. Send it to the person designated to review it according to your facility's policy.

Don't write *incident report completed* after charting the event. This destroys the confidential nature of the report and may result in a lawsuit. For the same reason, the doctor shouldn't write an order for an incident report in the chart.

In charting the incident, include everything the patient or family member says about his role in the incident. For example, you might write *Patient stated, "The nurse told me to ask for help before I went to the bathroom, but I decided to go on my own."* In a negligence lawsuit, this information may help the defense lawyer show that the incident was entirely or partially the patient's fault. If the jury finds that the patient was partially at fault, the concept of *contributory negligence* may be used to reduce or even eliminate the patient's recovery of damages.

Hazard #2: Informed consent

A patient must sign a consent form before most treatments and procedures. Informed consent means that he understands the proposed therapy and its risks and agrees to undergo it. The doctor performing the procedure is legally responsible for explaining the procedure and its risks and obtaining consent. However, he may ask you to witness the patient's signature. Some facilities may specifically require that the person who informs the patient of the treatment or procedure be the one to obtain the consent. Check with your facility's legal counsel if you have any questions. (See *Sign here: Witnessing a consent form.*)

Relinquishing requirements

The legal requirement for obtaining informed consent can be waived in only two situations:

☝ if a mentally competent patient says that he doesn't want to know the details of a treatment or procedure

✌ if an urgent medical or surgical situation occurs. (Many facilities specify how you should document such an emergency.)

Most facilities use a standard consent form that lists the legal requirements for consent. If the patient doesn't understand the doctor's explanation or asks for more information, answer all questions that fall within the scope of your practice. Be sure to document your interaction with the patient. (See *Informed consent,* page 224.)

Hazard #3: Advance directives

The Patient Self-Determination Act requires health care facilities to provide information about the patient's right to choose and refuse treatment. Facilities must also ask patients if they have advance directives, which are documents that state a patient's wishes regarding life-sustaining medical care in case the patient is no longer able to indicate his own wishes. Your job is to document that the patient received the required information and whether he

Advice from the experts

Sign here: Witnessing a consent form

After the doctor informs the patient about a medical procedure, he may ask you to obtain the patient's signature on the consent form and then sign as a witness. Before doing this, review the checklist below.

☐ Make sure that the patient is competent, awake, alert, and aware of what he's doing. He shouldn't be under the influence of alcohol, illicit drugs, or prescribed medications that impair his understanding or judgment.

☐ Ask the patient if the doctor explained the diagnosis, proposed treatment, and expected outcome to his satisfaction.

☐ Ask the patient if he's been told about the risks of the treatment or procedure, the possible consequences of refusing it, and alternative treatments or procedures.

☐ Ask the patient if he has any concerns or questions about his condition or the treatment. If he does, help him get answers from the doctor or other appropriate sources.

☐ Tell the patient that he can refuse the treatment without having other care or support withdrawn, and that he can withdraw his consent after giving it.

☐ Notify your nurse-manager and the doctor immediately if you suspect that the patient has doubts about his condition or the procedure, hasn't been properly informed, or has been coerced into giving consent. Performing a procedure without voluntary consent may be considered battery.

☐ Objectively document your assessment of the patient's understanding in the chart, noting the situation, his responses, and actions you took.

☐ When you're satisfied that the patient is well informed, have him sign the consent form including the date and time, and then sign your name as a witness.

☐ Remember that you're responsible for obtaining *oral* informed consent for any procedures that you'll be performing, such as inserting an I.V. line or a urinary catheter.

brought an advance directive with him. (See *Tips for dealing with advance directives*, page 225.)

When a patient's advance directive is given to the doctor, the nurse's orders may change, depending on the patient's wishes. For example, if the patient's family submits an advance directive for a patient on life support who does not want to be kept alive on a ventilator, the patient may be removed from the ventilator and comfort measures provided.

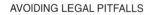

Art of the chart

Informed consent

If the patient signs a consent form, this implies that he understands the risks of a procedure and agrees to undergo it. Here's a typical form.

> The form should state the specific procedure under consideration.

CONSENT FOR OPERATION AND RENDERING OF OTHER MEDICAL SERVICES

1. I hereby authorize Dr. ____Wesley____ to perform upon ____Joseph Smith____ (Patient name), the following surgical and/or medical procedures: (State specific nature of the procedures to be performed) ____Exploratory laparotomy____

2. I understand that the procedure(s) will be performed at Valley Medical Center by or under the supervision of Dr. ____Wesley____, who is authorized to utilize the services of other doctors, or members of the house staff as he or she deems necessary or advisable.

3. It has been explained to me that during the course of the operation, unforeseen conditions may be revealed that necessitate an extension of the original procedure(s) or different procedure(s) than those set forth in Paragraph 1, I therefore authorize and request that the above named doctor, and his or her associates or assistants, perform such medical surgical procedures as are necessary and desirable in the exercise of professional judgment.

4. I understand the nature and purpose of the procedure(s), possible alternative methods of diagnosis or treatment, the possibility of complications, and the consequences of the procedure(s). I acknowledge th___ made as to the results that may be obtained.

> The patient acknowledges that he understands therapy and its risks and agrees to undergo it.

5. I authorize the above named doctor to administer local or regional anesthesia (for all other anesthesia manag___ sent must be signed by the patient or patient's authorized representative).

6. I understand that if it is necessary for me to receive a blood transfusion during this procedure or this hospitalization, the blood will be supplied by sources available to the hospital and tested in accordance with national and regional regulations. I understand that there are risks in transfusion, including but not limited to allergic, febrile, and hemolytic transfusion reactions, and the transmission of infectious diseases, such as hepatitis and AIDS (Acquired Immune Deficiency Syndrome). I hereby consent to blood transfusion(s) and blood derivative(s).

7. I hereby authorize representatives from Valley to photograph or videotape me for the purpose of research or medical education. It is understood and agreed that patient confidentiality shall be preserved.

8. I authorize the doctor named above and his or her associates and assistants and Valley Medical Center to preserve for scientific purposes or to dispose of any tissue, organs, or other body parts removed during surgery or other diagnostic procedures in accordance with customary medical practice.

9. I certify that I have read and fully understand the above consent statement. In addition, I have been afforded an opportunity to ask whatever questions I might have regarding the procedure(s) to be performed and they have been answered to my satisfaction.

____Joseph Smith____   ____11/15/97____   ____C. Gurney, RN____
Legal Patient or Authorized Representative   Date   Witness
(State Relationship to Patient)

If the patient is unable to consent on his or her own behalf, complete the following:

Patient _____ is unable to consent because _____

_____

Legally Responsible Person _____ Doctor Obtaining Consent ____M. Wesley, MD____

> Signing indicates only that you are witnessing the patient's signature.

The patient has the right to change advance directives at any time. Because the patient's requests may differ from what the family or doctor wants, document discrepancies carefully. (See *Check this out: Advance directive checklist,* page 227.)

Two common types of advance directives are:
- the living will
- the durable power of attorney for health care.

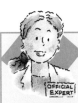

Advice from the experts

Tips for dealing with advance directives

Many patients wait until they're hospitalized to consider an advance directive or to make significant legal decisions. So, be prepared to offer information and advice and to record the patient's wishes in a legally appropriate manner. Here are some important points to remember.

Legal competence
Only a competent adult can execute a legally binding document. To prevent a patient's relatives from raising questions about his competence later, discuss his mental status with the doctor and, possibly, a psychiatrist. Be sure to document his mental status assessment in the chart *before* he signs any legal document.

Living will and durable power of attorney
If a patient has a living will or durable power of attorney for health care, a copy should be in his chart. Also, you should know how to contact the person with decision-making power. If the patient doesn't have the document with him, ask a family member to bring it to the health care facility. As your patient's advocate, you must ensure that his wishes are properly executed. If conflicts arise, discuss them with your nurse-manager and a risk manager.

If a patient wants to execute a living will during his hospital stay, you aren't required, or even allowed in some states, to sign as a witness. Many facilities have the social service or risk management department oversee this process. Find out who's responsible in your facility. The person who acts as witness can be held accountable for the patient's competence. Place the signed and witnessed document in the chart.

Last will and testament
In some facilities, dictating a patient's last will and testament is so commonplace that special forms have been designed for it. If this situation occurs often in your facility, discuss creating a form with your manager.

If no form exists in your facility, and a patient wants to dictate his last will and testament to you, document his request and what's been done to facilitate it; for example, who's been contacted and when.

If an administrator isn't available, two nurses should be present during dictation of the will. One should record the information in the chart, and both should sign it.

Living will

In making a living will, a legally competent person declares what medical care he wants or doesn't want if he develops a terminal illness. Living wills may apply only to treatment decisions made after a terminally ill patient becomes comatose and has no reasonable chance of recovery. They usually authorize the doctor to withhold or discontinue lifesaving measures.

> When the patient's wishes with regard to life-sustaining care clash with the doctor or family members, document the discrepancy.

Legal requirements

All states recognize living wills as valid legal documents. Although the legal requirements vary from state to state, most states specify:
• the circumstances under which a living will applies
• who is authorized to make a living will (usually only competent adults)
• limitations or restrictions on care that can be refused (for example, some states don't allow refusal of food and water)
• the elements the will must contain to be considered a legal document, including witnessing requirements
• who is immune from liability for following a living will's directions
• the procedure for rescinding a living will.

Durable power of attorney

A durable power of attorney for health care enables a person to state what type of care he does or doesn't want. However, it also names another person to make health care choices if the patient becomes legally incompetent. This person is usually a family member or friend or, in rare instances, the doctor.

Do-not-resuscitate policies

Do-not-resuscitate (DNR) orders are instructions not to attempt to resuscitate a patient who has suffered cardiac or respiratory failure. A DNR order may be appropriate if the patient has a terminal illness, is permanently unconscious, won't respond to cardiopulmonary resuscitation (CPR), or would be extraordinarily burdened by CPR. A terminally ill patient may ask not to be resuscitated if he experiences

Art of the chart

Check this out: Advance directive checklist

The JCAHO requires that information on advance directives be charted on the admission assessment form. However, many facilities also use a checklist like the one below.

ADVANCE DIRECTIVE CHECKLIST

Check appropriate boxes.

I. DISTRIBUTION OF ADVANCE DIRECTIVE INFORMATION

A. Advance directive information was presented to the patient: .... ☑

  1. At the time of preadmission testing .... ☑

  2. Upon inpatient admission .... ☐

  3. Interpretive services contacted .... ☐

  4. Information was read to the patient .... ☐

B. Advance directive information was presented to the next of kin as the patient is incapacitated .... ☐

C. Advance directive information was not distributed as the patient is incapacitated and no relative or next of kin was available .... ☐

<u>Mary Barren, RN</u>   <u>11/15/91</u>
RN   **DATE**

II. ASSESSMENT OF ADVANCE DIRECTIVE UPON ADMISSION

	Upon admission		Upon transfer to Critical Care Unit	
	YES	NO	YES	NO
A. Does the patient have an advance directive?	☐	☑	☐	☐
If yes, was the attending physician notified?	☐		☐	
B. If no advance directive, does the patient want to execute an advance directive?	☑	☐	☐	☐
If yes, was the attending physician notified?	☑		☐	
Was the patient referred to resources?	☑		☐	

Sign and date.

<u>Mary Barren, RN</u>   **RN**
RN
<u>11/15/91</u>
DATE   **DATE**

III. RECEIPT OF AN ADVANCE DIRECTIVE AFTER ADMISSION

A. The patient has presented an advance directive after admission and the attending physician has been notified.

Sign here if the patient has brought an advance directive and presented it after admission.

RN   **DATE**

sudden cardiac arrest, or he may write this request into his advance directive.

DNR orders should be reviewed periodically or whenever a significant change occurs in the patient's clinical status. (See *Charting last wishes.*)

If the patient doesn't ask for a DNR order, or if no policies exist, the doctor may write the order if it's medically appropriate and the patient understands the impact of the DNR order. If the patient is incompetent, an appropriate surrogate must give consent for the doctor to write the DNR order.

Hazard #4: Patients who refuse treatment

You're also responsible for helping patients make informed decisions about continuing treatment. When treatment is refused, important patient care, safety, and documentation issues come into play.

Refusing treatment

Any mentally competent adult can legally refuse treatment if he has been fully informed about his medical condition and the likely consequences of his refusal. This means he

Advice from the experts

Charting last wishes

Do-not-resuscitate (DNR) orders are extremely tricky. On the one hand, if a terminally ill patient asks not to be resuscitated, you must abide by his wishes if he goes into cardiac or respiratory arrest. Calling a code (initiation of emergency treatment by doctors and nurses to resuscitate a patient after cardiac or respiratory arrest) violates his right to refuse treatment. On the other hand, if you don't call a code, you could be accused of practicing medicine without a license and be found liable for his death.

Now what?
So how should you proceed? First, document the patient's wishes and chart his degree of awareness and orientation. Then contact your nurse-manager and request help from administration, legal services, or social services.

If the doctor knows about the patient's wish but still refuses to write a DNR order, document this in your notes. Like you, the doctor must abide by the patient's wishes and may be found liable if he doesn't. If the patient has prepared an advance directive, make sure that the doctor has seen it.

can refuse mechanical ventilation, tube feedings, antibiotics, fluids, and other treatments that are needed to keep him alive.

The patient who says "no"

When your patient refuses treatment, chart his exact words. Inform him of the risks involved in refusing treatment, preferably in writing. If he still refuses treatment, chart that you didn't provide the prescribed treatment, and then notify the doctor. The doctor will explain the risks to the patient again. If he continues to refuse treatment, the doctor will ask him to sign a refusal-of-treatment release form, which you may need to sign as a witness. (See *Witnessing refusal of treatment*, page 230.)

If the patient will not sign this form, document this, too. For extra protection, your facility may require you to have the patient's spouse or closest relative sign another refusal-of-treatment release form.

More and more facilities are informing patients soon after admission about their future treatment options. Discuss the patient's wishes at your first opportunity, and document the discussion in case he becomes incompetent later.

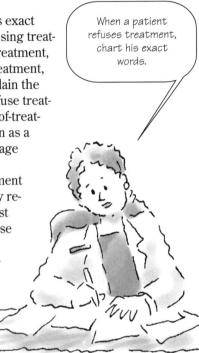

When a patient refuses treatment, chart his exact words.

Legal guidelines

Failure to respond appropriately to a patient's refusal to accept treatment may have serious legal consequences. To prevent problems, take these steps:
• Confirm the patient's condition and prognosis with the doctor and record them in the medical record.
• Make sure that the doctor documented the patient's understanding of the consequences of his refusal, such as pain or decreased life expectancy or quality of life.
• Search the medical record for a living will, a durable power of attorney for health care, or letters from people who heard the patient express his wishes.
• Search the medical record for documentation of conversations between the patient and health care providers, including the conversation about the patient's final decision to withhold treatment. Documentation should include the dates of conversations, the full names of people involved,

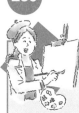

Art of the chart

Witnessing refusal of treatment

To prevent misunderstandings and lawsuits if a patient refuses treatment, the doctor must explain the risks involved in making this choice. If the patient still refuses treatment, the doctor will ask him to sign a refusal-of-treatment release form, such as the one below, which you may need to witness.

REFUSAL-OF-TREATMENT RELEASE FORM

> The patient acknowledges that he understands the risks of refusing treatment.

I, ___Joseph Arden___, refuse to allow anyone to ___administer parenteral nutrition___
   (patient's name)   (insert treatment)

The risks attendant to my refusal have been fully explained to me, and I fully understand the benefits of this treatment. I also understand that my refusal of treatment seriously reduces my chances for regaining normal health and may endanger my life.

I hereby release ___Memorial General___, its nurses and employees, together with all doctors in any way
                    (name of facility)
connected with me as a patient, from liability for respecting and following my express wishes and direction.

___Donna Burns___   ___Joseph Arden___
(Witness' signature)   (Patient's or legal guardian's signature)

___12/17/91___   ___16___
(Date)   (Patient's age)

---

the circumstances, and what treatments and medical conditions were discussed.
• DNR orders should be reviewed every 48 to 72 hours, or according to your facility's policy.
• DNR orders must be written; they cannot be provided as verbal orders or telephone orders.
• Refuse written or spoken orders for "slow codes." They may specify calling the doctor before resuscitating a patient, doing CPR but withholding drugs, giving oxygen but withholding CPR, or not putting a patient on a ventilator. These orders are unethical and illegal.

> Documentation to verify a patient's decision to withhold treatment must be handled carefully.

• Suggest that your facility set up an ethics committee to resolve problems about withholding treatment.

Hazard #5: Documenting for unlicensed personnel

Anyone reading your notes assumes these notes are a firsthand account of care provided — unless you chart otherwise. In some settings, nursing assistants and technicians aren't allowed to make formal chart entries. In such a case, determine what care was provided, assess the patient and the task performed (for example, a dressing change), and document your findings. Be sure to record the full names and titles of unlicensed personnel who provided care. Don't just record their initials.

If you are charting care provided by unlicensed personnel, assess the patient and the task performed and document your findings.

If your facility allows unlicensed personnel to chart, you may have to countersign their notes. If your facility's policy states that the person must provide care in your presence, don't countersign unless you actually witness her actions. If the policy says that you don't have to be there, your countersigning indicates that the notes describe care that other people had the authority and competence to perform and that you verified that the procedures were performed. You can specifically document that you reviewed the notes and consulted with the technician on certain aspects of care. Of course, you must document any follow-up care you provide.

Hazard #6: Using restraints

When physical restraints are ordered for a patient, your job is to check the patient frequently for problems associated with the restraints, perform range-of-motion exercises on all extremities, and then document your care. Most facilities have a policy outlining the proper procedure for using restraints. You may also recommend to the doctor that he order physical restraints for a patient and chart your observations in the progress notes. The doctor must reevaluate the need for physical restraints and rewrite orders for them every 24 hours. (See *Physical restraint order,* page 232.)

Art of the chart

Physical restraint order

A form such as the one below must be in the patient's chart before physical restraints are applied.

Date: _____11/2/91_____   Time: ____0315____

Reason for restraint use (circle all that apply):
To prevent:
    1. Falls
    2. Removal of indwelling lines/tubes ___(R) subclavian CV line___
    3. Self extubation
    4. Other _____

Duration of restraint: (Not to exceed 24 hr) ____24____

Type of restraint (circle all that apply):
    Vest
    Left mitt   Right mitt
    Left wrist   Right wrist
    Left ankle   Right ankle
    Other _____

Doctor's signature _____J. Donnelly, MD_____

If a competent patient refuses physical restraints, a facility may require him to sign a release absolving everyone involved of liability if he's injured as a result. (See *Charting the need for restraints.*)

Hazard #7: Patients who request to see their charts

A patient has a legal right to read his medical record. He may ask to see it because he's confused about the care he's receiving. First, ask him if he has questions about his treatment, and try to clear up any confusion.

If he still wants to see the record, check your facility's policy to see whether he has to read it in your presence. Document questions the patient asks about the record or statements he makes about it as well as what you say to him.

Art of the chart

Charting the need for restraints

The following progress note entry documents the need for restraints to ensure patient safety.

| 12/2/91 | 0100 | Pt found at 2345 holding onto ET tube and subclavian line and pulling at them. I explained the necessity of the ET tube and the subclavian line. At 0045 pt sleeping; ET tube and lines intact. ——————————————— Barbara Brogan, RN |
| 12/2/91 | 0200 | Pt again found pulling at ET tube. Dr. Smith notified. Left and right mitt restraints ordered. ——————————————— Barbara Brogan, RN |

Don't just hand it over

Never release medical records to unauthorized people, including family members and police officers. Refer all requests from insurance companies to the appropriate administrator, and refer other requests to your nurse-manager. Also notify her if you're in doubt about the validity of a request because she may want to notify the facility's administrator.

Hazard #8: Patients who leave against medical advice

The law says that a mentally competent patient can leave a facility at any time. Having the patient sign an against medical advice (AMA) form protects you, the doctors, and the facility if problems arise from his unapproved discharge.

Filling out the AMA form

The AMA form should clearly document that the patient knows he's leaving against medical advice, that he's been advised of and understands the risks of leaving, and that he knows he can come back. Use his own words to describe his refusal.

Here's what to include on the AMA form:
• the names of relatives or friends notified of the patient's decision and the dates and times of the notifications
• an explanation of the risks and consequences of the AMA discharge, as told to the patient, and the name of the person who provided the explanation
• other places the patient can go for follow-up care
• the names of people accompanying the patient at discharge and the instructions given to them
• the patient's destination after discharge.

If the patient leaves without anyone's knowledge, or if he refuses to sign the AMA form, check your facility's policy; you most likely have to fill out an incident report.

State the patient's state

In the progress notes, document statements and actions that reflect the patient's mental state at the time he left your facility. This helps protect you, the doctor, and the facility against a charge of negligence if the patient later claims that he was mentally incompetent at the time of discharge and was improperly supervised while in that state. (See *The patient's progress.*)

The case of the missing patient

Suppose a patient never says anything about leaving, but on rounds you discover he's missing. If you can't find him in the facility, notify your nurse-manager and the doctor; then try to contact the patient's home. If he's not there, call the police if you think the patient might hurt himself or others, especially if he left the hospital with any medical devices.

Chart the time you discovered the patient missing, your attempts to find him, the people you notified, and other pertinent information.

Art of the chart

The patient's progress

When a patient leaves against medical advice, document it in the progress notes, as shown below.

11/5/91	1300	Pt found in room dressed in own clothes with coat on. When asked why he was dressed, he stated, "They still don't know why I keep getting dizzy, and nothing is turning up in any of the tests. I don't want any more tests and I'm going home." Dr. McCarthy notified and came to speak with pt and his son. Pt willing to sign AMA form. AMA form signed. Pt told of the possible risks of his leaving the hospital with dizziness and hypertension. Pt agrees to see Dr. McCarthy in office tomorrow. Discussed appointment with pt and son. Pt going to son's home after discharge. Accompanied pt in wheelchair to main lobby with son. Pt left at 1245. ———————————— Lola Caudullo, RN

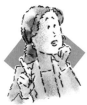

Quick quiz

1. Failure to provide patient care and to follow appropriate standards is called:
   A. breach of duty.
   B. breach of promise.
   C. negligent duty.

Answer: A. When investigating breach of duty, the courts ask: How would a reasonable, prudent nurse with comparable training and experience have acted in the same or similar circumstances?

2. Professional standards for most nursing specialties are set by:
   A. the court system.
   B. ANA.
   C. JCAHO.

Answer: B. ANA sets standards for most nursing specialities.

3. If you spill something on a page of the medical record, you should:
- A. throw the old page away after copying it.
- B. copy it and leave both pages in the chart.
- C. leave the stained page in the chart and write a note explaining what happened.

Answer: B. Discarding pages from the medical record, even for innocent reasons, will raise doubt in the jury's mind if the chart ends up in court.

4. If your facility uses flow sheets, checklists, and graphic forms, you still need to chart in the progress notes if:
- A. you filled out an incident report.
- B. there's any out-of-the-ordinary information.
- C. there are staff conflicts.

Answer: B. Anticipate litigation, and include in the progress notes anything that needs further explanation or clarification.

5. One way to expedite the charting process is to:
- A. ask another nurse to help with some of your charting.
- B. chart before you perform care, if you have more time then.
- C. chart your care as close to the time of the event as possible.

Answer: C. If you chart care right away, you'll be able to record it faster because events will be fresh in your mind.

Scoring

☆☆☆ If you answered all five items correctly, way to go! Document your achievement on an AMA (amazing meticulous attitude) form.

☆☆ If you answered three or four items correctly, terrific! Document your score on a DNR (definitely nice results) form.

☆ If you answered less than three correctly, don't worry. Draw a line through your test score, initial it, and try again.

Documenting procedures

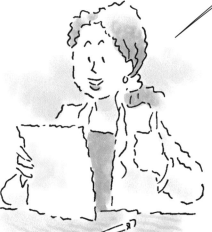

Just the facts

In this chapter, you'll learn:

◆ how to chart routine nursing procedures

◆ how to chart on a medication administration record

◆ extra steps to take when charting drug administration and I.V. therapy

◆ what to chart when you're assisting a doctor with a procedure.

Guidelines for charting nursing procedures

Your notes about routine nursing procedures usually appear in the patient's chart on flow sheets or graphic forms. Whatever your health care facility's requirements, you need to include this information in your documentation:
• what procedure was performed
• when it was performed
• who performed it
• how it was performed
• how well the patient tolerated it
• adverse reactions to the procedure, if any.

The section that follows outlines information that must be documented for several nursing procedures.

Take the time to document accurately, objectively, thoroughly, consistently, and legibly, both in routine and exceptional situations.

Drug administration

A medication administration record (MAR) is part of most documentation systems. It may be included in the medication Kardex, or it may be on a separate sheet. In either case, it's the central record of medication orders and their execution and is part of the patient's permanent record.

You chart MARvelously

When charting on the MAR, follow these guidelines:
- Obey your facility's policies and procedures for recording drug orders and administration.
- Record the patient's full name, the date, the drug's name, the dose, the administration route or method, the frequency, the number of doses given or the stop date (if applicable), and the administration time for doses given immediately. Also chart drug allergy information.
- Write legibly.
- Use only standard abbreviations. When in doubt, write out the word or phrase.
- After administering the first dose, sign your full name, licensure status, and initials in the appropriate space.
- Record drugs immediately after administering them so another nurse doesn't inadvertently repeat the dose.
- If you chart by computer, do it right after giving each drug — especially if you don't use printouts as a backup. This gives all team members access to the latest drug administration data.
- If a specific assessment parameter must be monitored during administration of a drug, document this requirement on the MAR. For example, when digoxin is administered, the patient's pulse rate needs to be monitored and this information needs to be charted on the MAR.
- If you didn't give a drug, document the reason.
- If you suspect that a patient's illness, injury, or death was drug-related, report this to the pharmacy department, who will relay the information to the Food and Drug Administration.

> Following these guidelines will help ensure safe drug administration.

P.r.n. medications

Chart all drugs administered as needed (p.r.n.).
- For eye, ear, or nose drops, chart the number of drops used and the administration route.
- For suppositories, chart the type (rectal, vaginal, or urethral) and how the patient tolerated it.

• For dermal drugs, chart the size and location of the area where you applied the drug and the condition of the skin or wound.
• For dermal patches, chart the location of the patch.
• For I.V., I.M., or S.C. medications, chart the dose given and the location of administration.

No room for exceptions

If you administer p.r.n. drugs according to accepted standards, you don't need to chart more specific information. However, if your MAR doesn't have space for exceptional data — such as a patient's response to a drug or refusal to take a drug — document this in the progress notes.

Drug abuse or refusal

If the patient refuses or abuses medications, describe the event in his chart. Here are some situations needing careful documentation:

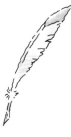

• You discover unprescribed drugs at the patient's bedside. Document the type of medication (pill or powder), the amount of medication, and its color and shape. (You may wish to send the drug to the pharmacy for identification.)
• You find a supply of prescribed drugs in the patient's bedside table, indicating that he isn't taking each dose. Record the type and amount of medication.
• You notice a sudden change in the patient's behavior after he has visitors, and you suspect them of giving him narcotics or other drugs. Document how the patient appeared before the visitors came and afterward.
• You offer prescribed medications and the patient refuses to take them. Document the refusal, the reason for it (if he tells you), and the medication. This prevents the refusal from being misinterpreted as an omission or a medication error on your part. Note the example below:

12/15/97	1100	Pt. refused K-Dur tabs, stating that they were too big and made her feel like she was choking when she tried to swallow one. Dr. Boyle notified. K-Dur tabs D/C. KCl elixir ordered and given. ——— Kathy Collins, RN

Report any medication abuse or refusal to the doctor. When you do so, document the name of the doctor and the date and time of notification.

Narcotic administration

Whenever you give a narcotic, you must document it according to federal, state, and facility regulations. These regulations require you to:
• sign out the drug on the appropriate form
• verify the amount of drug in the container before giving it
• have another nurse document your activity and observe you if you must waste or discard part of a narcotic dose
• count narcotics after each shift.

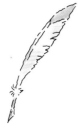

Two nurses should be present to count narcotic drugs — preferably the oncoming and offgoing nurse. If you discover a discrepancy in the narcotic count, report it, following your facility's policy. Also, file an incident report. An investigation will follow.

I.V. therapy

More than 80% of hospitalized patients receive some form of I.V. therapy, such as fluid or electrolyte replacement, total parenteral nutrition (TPN), drugs, or blood products. Document all facets of I.V. therapy carefully, including subsequent complications. Your facility may have you document in the progress notes, on a special I.V. therapy sheet or flowchart, or in another format.

Basic charting

After establishing an I.V. route, document the following information:
• the date, time, and venipuncture site
• the equipment used, such as the type and gauge of the catheter or needle
• the number of venipuncture attempts made and the type of assistance required (if applicable).
    Once per shift, document:
• the type, amount, and flow rate of I.V. fluid
• the condition of the I.V. site
• the fact that you flushed the I.V. line and what medication you used.
    Update your records each time you change the insertion site, venipuncture device, or I.V. tubing. Also docu-

ment the reason you changed the I.V. site, such as extravasation, phlebitis, occlusion, patient removal, or a routine change.

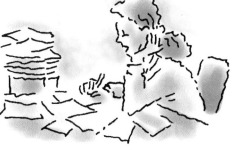

Each time I change the insertion site, venipuncture device, or tubing, I update my records.

Getting more involved

Document complications precisely. For example, record if extravasation occurs and what interventions you took, such as stopping the I.V., assessing the amount of fluid infiltrated, and notifying the doctor.

If a chemotherapeutic drug extravasates, stop the I.V. immediately and follow the procedure specified by the health care facility. Document the appearance of the I.V. site, the treatment you gave (especially antidotes), and the kind of dressing you applied. Document the amount of any discarded medication.

If the patient has an allergic reaction during I.V. therapy, stop the infusion and notify the doctor immediately. Then document all pertinent information about the reaction as well as your interventions and the patient's response.

Last but not least

Last, record patient and family teaching, such as explaining the purpose of I.V. therapy, describing the procedure itself, and discussing possible complications.

Total parenteral nutrition

If a patient is receiving TPN, document the type and location of the central line, the condition of the insertion site, and the volume and rate of the solution infused. When you discontinue a central or peripheral I.V. line for TPN, record the date and time, the type of dressing applied, and the appearance of the administration site.

Blood transfusions

Whenever you administer blood or blood components — such as packed cells, plasma, platelets, or cryoprecipitates — use proper identification and cross-matching procedures. Clearly document that you matched the label on the blood bag to:

- the patient's name
- the patient's medical record number
- the patient's blood group or type
- the patient's and donor's Rh factor
- the crossmatch data
- the blood bank identification number
- the expiration date of the product.

    In addition, the blood or blood component must be identified by two health care professionals, both of whom sign the slip that comes with the blood and verify that the information is correct.

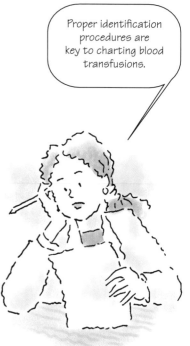

Proper identification procedures are key to charting blood transfusions.

For the record

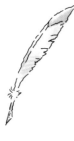

Once you determine that the information on the blood bag label is correct, you may administer the transfusion. Here's what to document on the transfusion record:

- the dates and times the transfusion was started and completed
- the name of the health care professional who verified the information
- the type and gauge of the catheter used
- the total amount of the transfusion
- the patient's vital signs before, during, and after the transfusion
- the infusion device used (if any) and its flow rate
- the blood warming unit used (if any).

Accounting for autotransfusions

If the patient receives his own blood, document the amount retrieved and reinfused in the intake and output records. Document the results of laboratory tests performed during and after the autotransfusion, paying special attention to the coagulation profile, hemoglobin and hematocrit values, and arterial blood gas and calcium levels. Also chart the patient's pretransfusion and posttransfusion vital signs.

Reacting to a transfusion reaction

If the patient develops a transfusion reaction, stop the transfusion immediately and notify the doctor. On a transfusion reaction form or in the progress notes, document the following:

- the time and date of the reaction
- the type and amount of infused blood or blood products

• the time you started and stopped the transfusion
• the clinical signs in order of occurrence
• the patient's vital signs per facility protocol
• whether urine specimens and blood samples were sent to the laboratory for analysis
• the treatment you gave and the patient's response to it.

You may need to send the uninfused blood back to the blood bank. An example of a note documenting a reaction is shown below.

11/16/91	1130	Pt reports nausea and chills. Transfusion started at 1030 hr. Cyanosis
		of the lips noted at 1100 hr with first unit of PRBCs transfusing.
		Stopped infusion. Approximately 100 ml infused. Tubing changed. I.V. of
		1,000 ml NSS infusing at 40 ml/hr in left hand. Dr. Dunn notified. BP
		170/90; P 110; R 28; T 99.4° F. Blood sample taken from PRBCs.
		Remaining blood discarded. Two red-top tubes of blood drawn from pt and
		sent to lab. Urine specimen obtained and sent to lab for UA. Pt given
		diphenhydramine 50 mg I.M. Two blankets placed on pt —— Anne Grasso, RN
	1145	Pt reports he's getting warmer and less nauseated. BP 164/86; P 100;
		R 24; T 99.2° F. ——————— Anne Grasso, RN
	1200	Pt without chills or nausea. I.V. 1,000 ml NSS infusing at 80 ml/hr in left
		hand. BP 156/82; P 92; R 22; T 98.9° F. ——— Anne Grasso, RN

Surgical incision care

When a patient returns from surgery, document his vital signs and level of consciousness and carefully record information about his surgical incision, drains, and the care you provide. An example of a progress note documenting surgical incision care is shown below.

11/17/91	1030	Dressing removed from right mastectomy incision; dime-sized area of serous
		sanguineous drainage on dressing. Incision well-approximated with staples
		intact. Site cleaned with sterile NSS. 4" x 4" sterile dressing applied.
		Teaching given to pt regarding dressing change and signs and symptoms of
		infection. Verbalized understanding. ——— Deborah Liu, RN

Records that get around

Also study the records that travel with the patient from the postanesthesia care unit. (See *Roaming records.*)

Look for a doctor's order stating whether you or he will perform the first dressing change. If you'll be performing it, document the following:

• the type of wound care performed
• the wound's appearance (size, color, condition of margins, and necrotic tissue); odor, if any; location of drains; and drainage characteristics (type, color, consistency, and amount)
• the type and amount of dressing and whether a pouch was applied
• additional wound care procedures, such as drain management, irrigation, and packing, or application of a topical medication
• how the patient tolerated the dressing change.

Detailed care and discharge data

In addition, document special or detailed wound care instructions and pain management measures on the nursing plan of care. Also chart the color and amount of measurable drainage on the intake and output form.

If the patient needs wound care after discharge, provide patient teaching and document it. Chart that you explained aseptic technique, described how to examine the wound for infection or other complications, demonstrated how to change the dressing, and gave written instructions for home care. Also document whether or not the patient demonstrates an understanding of the instructions and is able to perform wound care measures.

Pacemaker care

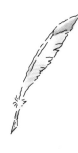

If the patient has a temporary pacemaker, record the following information:

• the date and time of placement
• the reason for placement
• pacemaker settings
• the patient's response
• the patient's level of consciousness (LOC) and vital signs, including which arm you used to obtain the blood pressure reading
• complications, such as chest pain or signs of infection
• interventions such as X-ray studies to verify correct electrode placement.

Advice from the experts

Roaming records

When your patient recovers from anesthesia, he'll be transferred from the operating room-postanesthesia care unit (OR-PACU) to his assigned unit for ongoing recovery and care. As his nurse, you're responsible for the four-part document that travels with the patient. Make sure the OR-PACU report is complete by checking for the following information.

Part 1: History
This section of the report should describe the patient's pertinent medical and surgical history, including drug allergies, medication history, chronic illnesses, significant surgical history, hospitalizations, and smoking history.

Part 2: Operation
This section describes the surgery itself and should include:
• the procedure performed
• the type and dosage of anesthetics
• how long the patient was anesthetized
• the patient's vital signs throughout surgery
• the volume of fluid lost and replaced
• drugs administered
• surgical complications
• tourniquet time
• drains, tubes, implants, or dressings used during surgery and removed or still in place.

Part 3: Postanesthesia period
This part of the record includes information about:
• pain medications and pain control devices that the patient received and how he responded to them
• interventions that should continue on the unit, such as frequent circulatory, motor, and neurologic checks if the patient underwent leg surgery and had a tourniquet on for a long time
• a flow sheet showing the patient's postanesthesia recovery scores on arrival and discharge in the areas of activity level, respiration, circulation, and level of consciousness (LOC).
• unusual events or complications that occurred on the OR-PACU; for example, nausea or vomiting, shivering, hypothermia, arrhythmias, central anticholinergic syndrome, sore throat, back or neck pain, corneal abrasion, tooth loss during intubation, swollen lips or tongue, pharyngeal or laryngeal abrasion, and postspinal headache.

Part 4: Current status
This section should describe the patient's status at the time of transfer back to the unit. Information should include his vital signs, LOC, and sensorium.

Make sure the rhythm strip includes the patient's name and the date and time of placement. An example of a progress note documenting pacemaker care is shown below.

12/1/97	1315	Pt with temporary transvenous pacemaker in
		right subclavian vein. Heart rate 60. Monitor
		showing 100% ventricular paced rhythm. ECG
		obtained. Pacemaker sensing and capturing
		correctly. Site without redness or swelling.
		Dressing dry and intact. —— Anne Salata, RN

If the patient has a transcutaneous pacemaker, document the reason for this kind of pacing, the time pacing started, and the locations of the electrodes.

You've got rhythm

Also document the information obtained from a 12-lead electrocardiogram (ECG). Put rhythm strips in the medical record before, during, and after pacemaker placement; any time pacemaker settings change; and any time the patient receives treatment for a pacemaker complication.

As ECG monitoring continues, record capture, sensing rate, intrinsic beats, and competition of paced and intrinsic rhythms.

Peritoneal dialysis

If your patient is receiving dialysis, monitor and document his response to treatment during and after the procedure. Here's what to chart:
• vital signs per facility protocol
• abrupt changes in the patient's condition and your notification of the doctor
• the amount of dialysate infused and drained and medications added (Complete a dialysis flowchart every 24 hours.)

• the effluent's characteristics and the assessed negative or positive fluid balance at the end of each infusion-dwell-drain cycle
• the patient's daily weight (immediately after the drain phase) and abdominal girth. Note the time of day and variations in the weighing and measuring technique.
• physical assessment findings
• fluid status
• equipment problems, such as kinked tubing or mechanical malfunction, and your interventions
• the condition of the patient's skin at the catheter site
• the patient's reports of unusual discomfort or pain and your interventions.

An example of a progress note documenting peritoneal dialysis is shown below.

12/20/91	0300	Pt receiving exchanges q2h of 1,500 ml 4.25 dialysate with 500 units
		heparin and 2 mEq, KCl; infused over 15 min. Dwell time 15 min. Drain
		time 30 min. Drainage clear, pale yellow fluid. Pt tolerating procedures
		without complications or discomfort. LLQ catheter site nonreddened.
		Site cleaned and dressed per protocol. Pt weight after dialysis 205 lb.
		Abdominal girth 45 1/2 ". ———————————— Amanda Taylor, RN

Peritoneal lavage

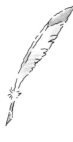

For the patient recovering from peritoneal lavage, document the following:
• vital signs and symptoms of shock, such as tachycardia, decreased blood pressure, diaphoresis, dyspnea, or vertigo
• the condition of the incision site
• the type and size of the peritoneal dialysis catheter used
• the type and amount of solution instilled into the peritoneal cavity
• the amount and color of the fluid withdrawn from the peritoneal cavity and whether it flowed freely in and out
• what specimens were obtained and sent to the laboratory for analysis
• complications that occurred and your interventions.

An example of a progress note documenting peritoneal lavage is shown below.

12/21/91	0400	#16 Fr. Foley catheter inserted without incident. NG tube inserted via right
		nostril to low intermittent suction. Dr. Byrne inserted # 15 Fr. peritoneal
		catheter below umbilicus via trocar; 20 ml clear fluid withdrawn. 750 ml warm
		NSS instilled as ordered and clamped. Pt turned from side to side. NSS dwell
		time 10 min, then drained freely from abdomen. Fluid samples sent to lab as
		ordered. Peritoneal catheter removed and incision closed by Dr. Byrne. 4" x 4"
		gauze pad with povidone-iodine ointment applied to site. Pt tolerated
		procedure well and is in no distress. ———————— Lois Testa, RN

Thoracic drainage

If your patient has thoracic drainage, record this information initially:
• the date and time the drainage began
• the type of system used
• the amount of suction applied to the pleural cavity
• the presence or absence of bubbling or fluctuation in the water-seal chamber
• the amount and type of drainage
• the patient's respiratory status.

At the end of each shift, record this information:
• how frequently you inspected the drainage system
• the presence or absence of bubbling or fluctuation in the water-seal chamber
• the patient's respiratory status
• the condition of the chest dressings
• the type, amount, and route of pain medication you gave
• complications and subsequent interventions.

The charting goes on and on

Ongoing documentation should include:
• the color, consistency, and amount of thoracic drainage in the collection chamber as well as the time and date of each observation

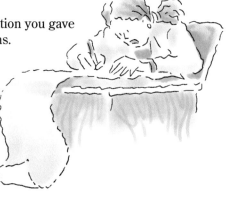

• patient-teaching sessions and activities you taught the patient to perform, such as coughing and deep breathing exercises, sitting upright, and splinting the insertion site to minimize pain
• the rate and quality of the patient's respirations and your auscultation findings
• complications, such as cyanosis, rapid or shallow breathing, subcutaneous emphysema, chest pain, or excessive bleeding, and the time and date you notified the doctor
• dressing changes and the patient's skin condition at the chest tube site.

An example of a progress note documenting thoracic drainage is shown below.

12/22/91	0100	Right anterior chest tube intact to 20 cm H₂O suction. 100 ml bright red bloody drainage noted since 0300. No air leak noted. + water chamber fluctuation. Chest tube site dressing dry and intact, no crepitus palpated. Resp. assessment unchanged as per flow sheet. ———————————— Nancy Siegfried, RN

Cardiac monitoring

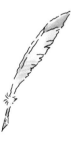

For the patient receiving cardiac monitoring, include the following information in your notes:
• the date and time that monitoring began
• the monitoring leads used
• rhythm strip readings labeled with the patient's name and room number and the date and time
• changes in the patient's condition.

An example of a progress note documenting cardiac monitoring is shown on the next page.

```
12/24/97 | 1315 | At 1245 monitor showing ST (HR 150s)
         |      | with multifocal PVCs. Pt complaining of
         |      | SOB and palpitations. O₂ 2 L via nasal
         |      | cannula placed. BP 178/96. ECG done.
         |      | Dr. Corcoran notified and he administered
         |      | Lopressor 5 mg I.V. at 1250. Blood drawn
         |      | for serum electrolytes and sent to lab.
         |      | Monitor presently showing NSR with
         |      | occasional multifocal PVCs. Pt without
         |      | SOB, chest pain, or palpitations at present.
         |      |                        —— Nancy Ghwan, RN
```

Keep on chartin'

If the patient will continue cardiac monitoring after discharge, document the following:
• which caregivers can interpret dangerous rhythms and perform cardiopulmonary resuscitation
• patient and family teaching, including troubleshooting techniques to use if the monitor malfunctions
• referrals to equipment suppliers, home health agencies, and other community resources.

Chest physiotherapy

Whenever you perform chest physiotherapy, document the following:
• the date and time of your interventions
• the patient's positions for secretion drainage and how long he remains in each
• the chest segments you percussed or vibrated
• the characteristics of the secretion expelled, including color, amount, odor, viscosity, and the presence of blood
• the patient's tolerance of the chest physiotherapy
• complications and your interventions.

An example of a progress note documenting chest physiotherapy is shown on the next page.

12/28/97	1130	Pt placed on right side of bed in
		Trendelenburg position. Chest physiotherapy
		and postural drainage performed for 10 min
		from lower to middle then upper lobes as
		ordered. Productive cough produced large
		amount yellow tenacious sputum. Pt tolerated
		procedure without difficulty; lungs clear to
		auscultation. ———————— Harry Moppert, RN

Mechanical ventilation

For patients receiving mechanical ventilation, chart this information initially:
• the date and time that mechanical ventilation began
• the type of ventilator used and its settings
• the patient's responses to mechanical ventilation, including vital signs, breath sounds, use of accessory muscles, secretions, intake and output, and weight.

Keep on chartin'

Throughout mechanical ventilation, chart this information:
• complications and subsequent interventions
• pertinent laboratory data, including results of arterial blood gas (ABG) analyses and oxygen saturation findings
• the duration of spontaneous breathing and the ability to maintain the weaning schedule for patients receiving pressure support ventilation or those using a T-piece or tracheostomy collar
• the rate of controlled breaths, the time of each breath rate reduction, and the rate of spontaneous respirations for patients receiving intermittent mandatory ventilation, with or without pressure support ventilation
• adjustments made in ventilator settings as a result of ABG levels
• adjustments of ventilator components, such as draining condensate into a collection trap and changing, cleaning, or discarding the tubing
• interventions to increase mobility, protect skin integrity, or enhance ventilation; for example, active or passive

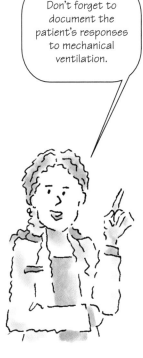

Don't forget to document the patient's responses to mechanical ventilation.

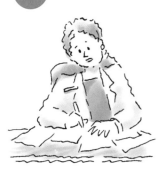

range-of-motion exercises, turning, or positioning the patient upright for lung expansion
• assessment findings related to peripheral circulation, urine output, decreased cardiac output, fluid volume excess, or dehydration
• the patient's sleep and wake periods, noting significant trends
• patient and family teaching in preparation for the patient's discharge, especially that associated with ventilator care and settings, artificial airway care, communication, nutrition, and therapeutic exercise
• teaching discussions and demonstrations related to signs and symptoms of infection and equipment functioning
• referrals to equipment vendors, home health agencies, and other community resources.

An example of a progress note documenting mechanical ventilation is shown below.

12/29/91	1100	ventilator wean started, placed 40%
		T-piece from 0930 to 1030. O_2 sat.
		remained above 90% during the entire
		weaning period. Resp. assessment unchanged
		from flow sheet; pt in no distress at present.
		———————————— John Devine, RN

Nasogastric tube insertion and removal

After you insert a nasogastric (NG) tube, record this information:
• the type and size of the NG tube
• the date, time, and insertion route (left nare, right nare, oral)
• the type and amount of suction
• the amount, color, consistency, and odor of the drainage
• how the patient tolerated the insertion procedure
• signs and symptoms of complications, such as nausea, vomiting, and abdominal distention

• subsequent irrigation procedures and problems occurring afterward, if any.

Record information about irrigations on an input and output sheet. An example of a progress note documenting NG tube replacement is shown below.

12/30/91	2100	#12 Fr. NG tube placed in right nare.
		Placement verified and tube attached to
		low intermittent suction, as ordered. Drainage
		dark brown; heme +. Dr. Cohen notified.
		Hypoactive bowel sounds in all 4 quadrants.
		Pt tolerated procedure well. —————
		————————————— Diane Harris, RN

Just a few more details

After you remove an NG tube, record the following:
• the date and time of removal
• how the patient tolerated the procedure
• unusual events accompanying tube removal, such as nausea, vomiting, abdominal distention, and food intolerance.

Seizure management

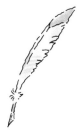

If your patient had a seizure while hospitalized, document this information:
• what seizure precautions you took
• the date and time that a seizure began and its duration
• precipitating factors, including aura-like sensations
• involuntary behavior occurring before the seizure, such as lip smacking, chewing movements, or hand and eye movements
• incontinence during the seizure
• the patient's vital signs (response to the seizure)
• what medications you gave
• complications resulting from the medications or the seizure and your interventions
• your assessment of the patient's postseizure mental status.

An example of a progress note documenting seizure management is shown below.

12/30/91	1615	At 1500 pt observed with generalized tonic-clonic seizure activity lasting 3 min. Awake at time of onset and stated, "Here it comes!" + urinary incontinence during seizure. Siderail pads in place prior to seizure. Placed on left side, airway patent. Dr. Defabio notified of seizure. Diazepam 10 mg given I.V. as ordered. Pt sleeping at present. Vital signs stable (see graphic form). No further seizure activity noted.————Barbara Chao, RN

Suture removal

Usually, the doctor will write an order for you to remove sutures alone. When documenting this procedure, record:
• the date and time the sutures were removed
• the appearance of the suture line
• the appearance of the wound site, including the presence of purulent drainage
• if and when you notified the doctor
• if and when you collected a specimen and sent it to the laboratory for analysis.

Tube feedings

When documenting your care of a patient receiving tube feedings, write down:
• the patient's tolerance of the procedure and the feeding formula
• the kind of tube feeding the patient is receiving (such as duodenal or jejunal feedings or a continuous drip or bolus)
• the amount, rate, route, and method of feeding (with continuous feedings, document the rate hourly)
• the dilution strength if you need to dilute the formula (for example, half-strength or three-quarters strength)
• the time you flushed the tube and the solution used (if applicable)

• the time you replaced the tube and how the patient tolerated the procedure (if applicable)
• a description of the patient's gastric function, including prescribed medications or treatments to relieve constipation or diarrhea
• urine and serum glucose, serum electrolyte, and blood urea nitrogen levels, as well as serum osmolality values
• feeding complications, such as hyperglycemia, glycosuria, and diarrhea
• patient and family teaching if the patient will continue receiving tube feedings after discharge
• referrals to suppliers or support agencies.

Obtaining an arterial blood sample

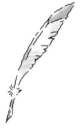

When you must obtain blood for ABG analysis, record the following:
• the patient's vital signs and temperature
• the arterial puncture site
• the results of Allen's test
• indications of circulatory impairment, such as swelling, discoloration, pain, numbness, or tingling in the bandaged arm or leg, and bleeding at the puncture site
• the time you drew the blood sample
• how long you applied pressure to the site to control bleeding
• the type and amount of oxygen therapy that the patient was receiving (if applicable).

An example of a progress note documenting obtainment of an arterial blood sample is shown below.

12/31/91	0930	Blood drawn from left radial artery after + Allen's
		test, brisk capillary refill. Pressure applied to
		site for 5 min and pressure dressing applied.
		No swelling, bleeding, or hematoma noted.
		Hand pink and warm, with brisk capillary
		refill. Dr. Smith notified of ABG results; O₂
		increased to 40% nonrebreather mask at
		0845. Pt in no resp. distress. ————
		—————— Karen Andrews, RN

Surprise! Another form

When filling out a laboratory request form for ABG analysis, include the following information:
• the patient's current temperature and respiratory rate
• his most recent hemoglobin level
• the fraction of inspired oxygen and tidal volume if he's receiving mechanical ventilation.

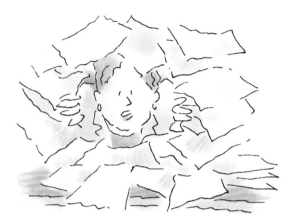

Charting assistive procedures

When you assist a doctor during a procedure, your role is also to provide patient support and teaching, to evaluate the patient's response, and to document the procedure carefully. Regardless of the procedure, you must always document the following:
• the date, time, and name of the procedure
• the doctor who performed it
• how it was performed
• how the patient tolerated it
• adverse reactions to the procedure, if any.
The section that follows describes documentation for several assistive procedures.

Bone marrow aspiration

After assisting the doctor with bone marrow aspiration, document the following:
• the date and time of the procedure
• the name of the doctor performing the procedure
• the appearance of the specimen aspirated
• how the patient responded to the procedure
• the location and appearance of the aspiration site, including bleeding and drainage
• the patient's vital signs after the procedure.

An example of a progress note documenting assistance during bone marrow aspiration is shown on the next page.

12/3/91	1015	Bone marrow aspiration explained to patient
		with questions answered. Bone marrow
		aspiration on left iliac crest performed by
		Dr. Wallace at 0945. No bleeding at site.
		Specimens sent to lab as ordered. Main-
		taining bed rest. Vital signs stable. Pt
		tolerated procedure well. Pamela Clark, RN

Esophageal tube insertion and removal

After assisting with esophageal tube insertion or removal, document the following:

• the date and time that you assisted in the insertion or removal

• the name of the doctor who performed the procedure

• the intragastric balloon pressure, the amount of air injected into the gastric balloon port, the amount of fluid used for gastric irrigation, and the color, consistency, and amount of gastric return both before and after lavage (if applicable)

• the baseline intraesophageal balloon pressure, which varies with respirations and esophageal contractions

• the patient's tolerance of both the insertion and removal procedures.

• vital signs before, during, and after the procedure.

An example of a progress note documenting esophageal tube insertion is shown below.

11/4/91	1320	Sengstaken-Blakemore tube placed without difficulty by Dr. Weathers via
		left nare. 50 cc air injected into gastric balloon, then 500 cc air
		injected into gastric balloon after abdominal X-ray confirmed placement. Tube
		secured to football helmet traction. Large amount of bright red blood drainage
		noted. Tube irrigated with 1,800 ml of iced NSS until clear. Esophageal
		balloon inflated to 30 mm Hg and clamped. Vital signs stable. Equal breath
		sounds bilat. Pt tolerated procedure well. Emotional support given.————
		———————————————————————— James Carr, RN

Arterial line insertion and removal

When assisting the doctor who's inserting an arterial line, record:
- the date and time
- the doctor's name
- the insertion site
- the type, gauge, and length of the catheter
- the patient's response to the procedure.

An example of a progress note documenting insertion of an arterial line is shown below.

11/5/91	0820	20G arterial catheter placed in left radial
		artery by Dr. Watson after + Allen's test.
		Transducer leveled and zeroed. Readings
		accurate to cuff pressures. Site without
		redness, swelling, or ecchymosis. Dressed
		as per protocol. Left hand and wrist taped
		and secured to armboard. Line flushes easily.
		Arterial waveform visible on monitor. Hand
		warm and pink with brisk capillary refill. ——
		—————————————————— Harry Nguen, RN

Now, record removal

After removing the arterial line, record:
- the date and time
- the doctor's name
- the length of the catheter
- the condition of the insertion site
- specimens that were obtained from the catheter for culture
- the patient's response to the procedure.

Central venous line insertion and removal

When you help the doctor insert a central venous (CV) line, you need to document:
- the time and date of insertion
- the doctor's name

- the length and location of the catheter
- the solution infused
- the patient's response to the procedure
- the time that X-rays were done to confirm correct placement, the results, and when you notified the doctor of them. Also document if more than one attempt was made to insert the catheter.

An example of a progress note documenting insertion of a central venous line is shown below.

11/6/91	1030	Procedure explained to pt and consent obtained by Dr. Rafferty.
		Triple-lumen catheter placed by Dr. Rafferty on 2nd attempt in left subclavian.
		Catheter sutured in place and dressing applied as per protocol. All lines
		flushed with 5 ml NSS. Portable chest X-ray obtained to confirm placement. Pt
		tolerated procedure well. Vital signs stable. ————————Eva Ryan, R.N.

Again, record removal

After assisting with removal of a CV line, record:
- the time and date of removal
- the type of dressing applied
- the condition of the insertion site
- catheter specimens you collected for culture or other analysis.

Lumbar puncture

During a lumbar puncture, observe the patient closely for signs of complications, such as a change in LOC, dizziness, or changes in vital signs. Report these to the doctor immediately and document them carefully. Also document the following:
- the color and clarity of the fluid obtained
- the number of test tubes sent to the lab for analysis
- how the patient tolerated the procedure
- observations about the patient's condition and your interventions, including keeping him in a supine position for 6 to 12 hours, encouraging fluid intake, and assessing for headache and leaking CSF around the puncture site.

Paracentesis

When caring for a patient during and after paracentesis, document the following information:
• the date and time of the procedure
• the puncture site
• whether or not the site was sutured
• the amount, color, viscosity, and odor of the initially aspirated fluid (also record this in the intake and output record).

If you're responsible for ongoing patient care, also document:
• a running record of the patient's vital signs
• the frequency of drainage checks per facility protocol
• the patient's response to the paracentesis
• the characteristics of the drainage, including color, amount, odor, and viscosity
• the patient's daily weight and abdominal girth measurements (taken at about the same time every day)
• what fluid specimens were sent to the laboratory for analysis
• peritoneal fluid leakage, if any. (Be sure to notify the doctor and chart the time and date.)

An example of a progress note documenting paracentesis is shown below.

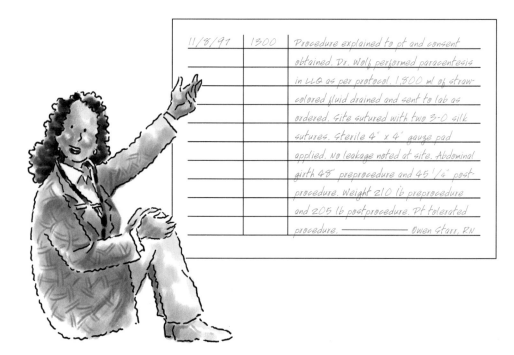

11/8/91	1300	Procedure explained to pt and consent
		obtained. Dr. Wolf performed paracentesis
		in LLQ as per protocol. 1,800 ml of straw-
		colored fluid drained and sent to lab as
		ordered. Site sutured with two 3-0 silk
		sutures. Sterile 4" x 4" gauze pad
		applied. No leakage noted at site. Abdominal
		girth 48" preprocedure and 45 1/4" post-
		procedure. Weight 210 lb preprocedure
		and 205 lb postprocedure. Pt tolerated
		procedure. ————— Owen Starr, RN

Thoracentesis

When assisting with thoracentesis, chart this information:
• the date and time of the procedure
• the name of the doctor who performed it
• the amount and characteristics of fluid aspirated
• the patient's response to the procedure
• if the patient had sudden or unusual pain, faintness, dizziness, or changes in vital signs, and when you reported these problems to the doctor
• symptoms of pneumothorax, hemothorax, subcutaneous emphysema, or infection; when you reported them to the doctor; and your interventions
• when you sent a fluid specimen to the laboratory for analysis.

An example of a progress note documenting thoracentesis is shown below.

11/10/91	1100	Procedure explained to pt and consent obtained
		by Dr. McCall. Pt positioned over secured
		bedside table. RLL thoracentesis performed
		by Dr. McCall without incident. Sterile
		4" x 4" gauze dressing applied to site; site
		without redness, edema, or drainage. 900 ml
		straw-colored fluid aspirated and specimens
		sent to lab as ordered. Vital signs stable.
		Lungs clear to auscultation. ————
		————Donna Taylor, RN

Charting miscellaneous procedures

Documentation isn't limited to procedures you perform yourself or help the doctor perform. You'll also chart in other situations, including the ones described below.

Diagnostic tests

Before receiving a diagnosis, most patients undergo testing, which can be as simple as a blood test or as complicated as magnetic resonance imaging. Record in the medical record all tests and how the patient tolerated them.

Chart your first impressions

Start your documentation by recording preliminary assessments you made of the patient's condition. For example, chart if she's pregnant or has allergies, because these conditions might affect the way a test is performed or the test's result. If the patient's age, illness, or disability requires special preparation for a test, record this information as well.

Also chart what you taught the patient about the test and follow-up care, the administration or withholding of drugs and preparations, special diets, food or fluid restrictions, enemas, and specimen collection.

An example of a progress note documenting a diagnostic test is shown below.

> When charting a diagnostic test, begin by recording your preliminary assessment findings.

11/13/91	0600	24-hr test for urine protein started. Pt instructed on purpose of test and how to collect urine. Demonstrated correct technique. Sign placed on pt's door and in bathroom. Specimen container placed on ice in bathroom. ———— Mary Brady, RN

Pain control

In your quest to eliminate or minimize your patient's pain, you may use a number of assessment tools to determine the degree of pain. When you use these tools, always document the results. (See *Chart pain three ways*.)

When charting pain levels and characteristics, determine whether the pain is internal, external, localized, or diffuse, and whether it interferes with the patient's sleep or other activities of daily living. Describe the pain in the patient's own words and enter them in the chart.

Art of the chart

Chart pain three ways

Some facilities use standardized questionnaires, such as the McGill-Melzack Pain Questionnaire or the Initial Pain Assessment Tool. But if your facility doesn't, you can devise your own pain measurement tools, such as the flow sheet and rating scales shown below. Whichever pain assessment tool you choose, remember to document its use and put the graphic form in your patient's chart.

Pain flow sheet

Flow sheets are convenient tools for pain assessment because they allow you to reevaluate the patient's pain at regular intervals. They're also useful when patients and families feel too overwhelmed to answer a long, detailed questionnaire.

Try to incorporate pain assessment into the flow sheet you're already using. The easier it is to use the flow sheet, the more likely you and your patient will be to use it.

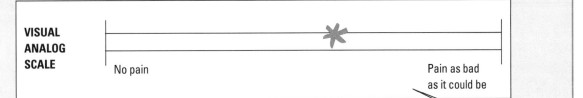

PAIN FLOW SHEET

Record the patient's pain before medication administration here.

Record the patient's pain after medication administration here.

...nd	Pain rating (0 to 10)	Patient behaviors	Vital signs	Pain rating after intervention	Comments
...0/91 0800	1	Wincing; holding head	BP 186/188 HR 98 - RR 22	5	Dilaudid 2 mg I.M. given
11/20/91 1200	3	Relaxing; reading	BP 160/80 HR 84 - RR 18	2	

Visual analog pain scale

In a visual analog pain scale, the patient marks a linear scale at the point that corresponds to his perceived degree of pain. The typical scale shown below uses the phrases "no pain" at one end and "pain as bad as it could be" at the other end.

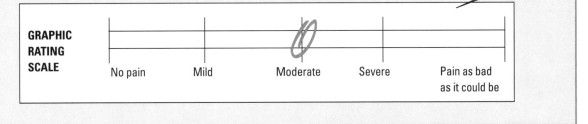

VISUAL ANALOG SCALE

No pain ———————————————————— Pain as bad as it could be

The patient fills out these forms.

Graphic rating scales

Graphic rating scales are similar to visual analog scales, but they show more degrees of pain intensity. Have the patient mark the spot on the continuum that best describes his pain.

GRAPHIC RATING SCALE

No pain | Mild | Moderate | Severe | Pain as bad as it could be

Paying attention to body language

Be aware of the patient's body language and behaviors associated with pain. Does he wince or grimace? Does he move or squirm in bed? What positions seem to relieve or worsen the pain? What other measures — such as heat, cold, massage, or drugs — relieve or heighten the pain? Also note if the pain appears to worsen or improve when visitors are present. Document all of this information as well as your interventions and how the patient responded.

An example of a progress note documenting care for a patient with pain is shown below.

| 12/22/91 | 0800 | Pt admitted with osteosarcoma and severe lower back pain. Took ibuprofen 800 mg q6h at home without relief last night or this morning. Dr. Kobb notified. Morphine 2 mg ordered and given I.V. at 0715. Vital signs stable. Pt states relief given. ———————— Sarah Bane, RN |

Intake and output

Many patients, including surgical and burn patients, those receiving I.V. therapy, and those with fluid and electrolyte imbalances, hemorrhage, or edema need 24-hour intake and output monitoring. To expedite documentation, you'll probably keep intake and output sheets at the bedside or by the bathroom door. If the patient is incontinent, document this as well as tube drainage and irrigation volumes.

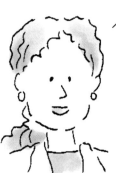

Keeping track of intake requires the cooperation of the patient and colleagues.

The intake charting challenge

Keeping track of foods and fluids that are premeasured is easy. You can list the volumes of specific containers for quick reference and also use infusion devices to more accurately record enteral and I.V. intake.

Keeping track of intake that isn't premeasured is harder. For example, measuring and recording a food like gelatin that's fluid at room temperature requires the cooperation of the patient and other caregivers. You'll also need to teach family members and friends to record or report to you all snacks and soft drinks they bring the patient and all meals they help him eat.

Don't forget these types of intake

Don't forget to document as intake I.V. piggyback infusions, drugs given by I.V. push, patient-controlled analgesics, and irrigation solutions that aren't withdrawn. Also chart oral or I.V. fluids that the patient receives when he's not on your unit. This requires the cooperation of the patient and staff members in other departments. In addition, remind ambulatory patients to use a urinal or a commode.

Fluid loss through the GI tract is normally 100 ml or less daily. However, if the patient's stools become excessive or watery, you must document them as output. Vomiting, drainage from suction devices and wound drains, and bleeding are other measurable sources of fluid loss that require documentation.

Codes

Guidelines established by the American Heart Association direct you to keep a written, chronological account of a patient's condition throughout CPR. If you're the designated recorder, document therapeutic interventions and the patient's responses *as* they occur. Don't rely on your memory later.

The form used to chart a code is the *code record*. It incorporates detailed information about your observations and interventions as well as drugs given to the patient. (See *Charting CPR*, page 266.)

Some facilities use a *resuscitation critique form* to identify actual or potential problems with the resuscitation process. This form tracks personnel responses and response times as well as the availability of appropriate drugs and functioning equipment.

> During CPR, the designated recorder should document events as they occur.

Art of the chart

Charting CPR

A completed code record like the one below should be included in your patient's chart.

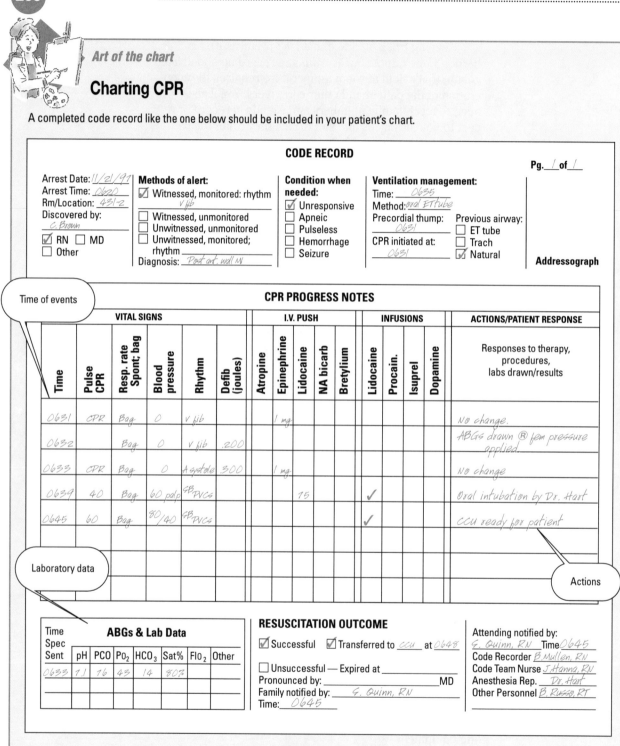

CODE RECORD

Pg. _1_ of _1_

Arrest Date: _11/21/97_
Arrest Time: _0620_
Rm/Location: _431-2_
Discovered by: _C. Brown_
☑ RN ☐ MD
☐ Other

Methods of alert:
☑ Witnessed, monitored: rhythm _v. fib_
☐ Witnessed, unmonitored
☐ Unwitnessed, unmonitored
☐ Unwitnessed, monitored; rhythm
Diagnosis: _Post ant. wall MI_

Condition when needed:
☑ Unresponsive
☐ Apneic
☐ Pulseless
☐ Hemorrhage
☐ Seizure

Ventilation management:
Time: _0635_
Method: _oral ET tube_
Precordial thump: _0631_
CPR initiated at: _0631_

Previous airway:
☐ ET tube
☐ Trach
☑ Natural

Addressograph

Time of events

CPR PROGRESS NOTES

	VITAL SIGNS						I.V. PUSH					INFUSIONS				ACTIONS/PATIENT RESPONSE
Time	Pulse CPR	Resp. rate Spont; bag	Blood pressure	Rhythm	Defib (joules)	Atropine	Epinephrine	Lidocaine	NA bicarb	Bretylium	Lidocaine	Procain.	Isuprel	Dopamine	Responses to therapy, procedures, labs drawn/results
0631	CPR	Bag	0	V fib			1 mg								No change.
0632		Bag	0	V fib	.200										ABGs drawn ® fem pressure applied.
0633	CPR	Bag	0	A systole	300		1 mg								No change
0639	40	Bag	60 palp	SB PVCs				15			✓				Oral intubation by Dr. Hart
0645	60	Bag	80/40	SB PVCs							✓				CCU ready for patient

Laboratory data

Actions

Time Spec Sent	ABGs & Lab Data						
	pH	PCO₂	Po₂	HCO₃	Sat%	FIo₂	Other
0633	7.1	16	43	14	80%		

RESUCITATION OUTCOME

☑ Successful   ☑ Transferred to _CCU_ at _0648_

☐ Unsuccessful — Expired at _____
Pronounced by: _____ MD
Family notified by: _G. Quinn, RN_
Time: _0645_

Attending notified by:
G. Quinn, RN Time _0645_
Code Recorder _B. Mullen, RN_
Code Team Nurse _J. Hanna, RN_
Anesthesia Rep. _Dr. Hart_
Other Personnel _B. Russo, RT_

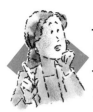

Quick quiz

1. When using an MAR, you need to:
   A. use abbreviations that only people on your unit understand.
   B. squeeze in as much information as possible.
   C. record drugs immediately after you give them.

Answer: C. This prevents other nurses from inadvertently giving the drug again.

2. After you establish an I.V. route, document:
   A. each time you check the I.V. setup.
   B. the condition of the patient's veins.
   C. the number of venipuncture attempts if more than one is made.

Answer: C. Chart the number of attempts you made and the type of assistance required.

3. In charting about mechanical ventilation, include:
   A. only the ventilator adjustments you make.
   B. your assessment findings.
   C. only the patient's objective responses.

Answer: B. Document assessment findings related to peripheral circulation, urine output, decreased cardiac output, fluid volume excess, or dehydration.

4. When assisting a doctor with procedures, document:
   A. only what you did yourself.
   B. why you think the patient is having the procedure done.
   C. the doctor's name and the patient's response.

Answer: C. Also record the date and time, pertinent information about the procedure, the patient's response, and your patient teaching.

5. Before giving a blood transfusion:
   A. ask another health professional to identify and document the blood or blood component.
   B. ask the patient if he'd rather receive his own blood.
   C. try to figure out if he'll develop a reaction.

Answer: A. You also need to match the patient's name, medical record number, blood group or type, Rh factor (patient's and donor's), crossmatch data, and blood bank identification number with the label on the blood bag — and then document that you did so.

6. A tool for documenting pain is the:
   A. French scale.
   B. Graphic rating scale.
   C. analogous graphic sheet.

Answer: B. This tool allows the patient to chart his degree of pain on a linear scale.

Scoring

☆☆☆   If you answered all six items correctly, gadzooks! You're able to complete tall stacks of medical records in a single round!

☆☆   If you answered four or five correctly, leaping lizards! You've performed your purpose: polishing off a plethora of paperwork!

☆   If you answered fewer than four correctly, don't worry! You can go back and review this chapter, take this book to work, and feel confident knowing you have a reference that makes charting incredibly easy.

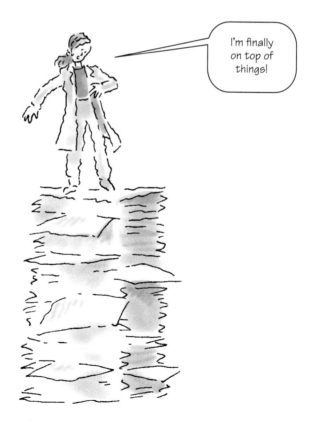

Glossary and index

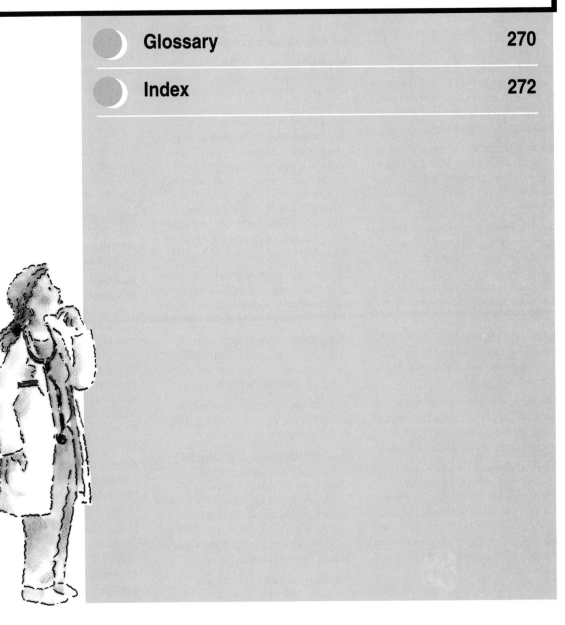

Glossary

Accountability: obligation to accept responsibility for or account for one's actions

Accreditation: official recognition from a professional or government organization that a health care facility meets relevant standards

Advance directive: document used as a guideline for life-sustaining medical care of a patient with an advanced disease or disability, who is no longer able to indicate his own wishes; includes living wills and durable powers of attorney for health care

Barthel index and scale: functional assessment tool used to evaluate an older patient's overall well-being and self-care abilities; evaluates the ability to perform 10 self-care activities

Case management: model for management of health care facilities in which one professional — usually a nurse or a social worker — assumes responsibility for coordinating care so that patients move through the health care system in the shortest time and at the lowest cost possible

Charting by exception (CBE): charting system that departs from traditional systems by requiring documentation of only significant or abnormal findings

Core charting: charting system that focuses on the nursing process; components include a database, plan of care, flow sheets, progress notes, and discharge summary

Critical pathway: documentation tool used in managed care and case management in which a time line is defined for the patient's condition and for the achievement of expected outcomes; used by caregivers to determine on any given day where the patient should be in his progress toward optimal health

Database: subjective and objective patient information collected during your initial assessment of the patient; includes information obtained by taking your patient's health history, performing a physical examination, and analyzing laboratory test results

Diagnosis-related group (DRG): system of classifying or grouping patients according to medical diagnosis for purposes of reimbursement of hospitalization costs under Medicare (For example, according to the DRG system, all patients admitted to the hospital for a surgical procedure, such as coronary bypass, would be eligible for the same reimbursement from Medicare regardless of actual cost to the hospital. If the patient's hospital bill should total less than the amount paid by Medicare regardless of actual cost to the hospital, the hospital is allowed to keep the difference.)

Durable power of attorney for health care: Legal document whereby a patient authorizes another person to make medical decisions for him should he become incompetent to do so

Focus charting: charting system that uses assessment data, first to evaluate patient-centered topics (or foci of concern) and then to document precisely and concisely

Health history: summary of a patient's health status that includes physiologic, psychological, cultural, and psychosocial data

Health maintenance organization (HMO): organization that provides an agreed-upon health service to voluntary enrollees who prepay a fixed, periodic fee that is set without regard to the amount or kind of services received (People who belong to an HMO are cared for by member doctors with limited referrals to outside specialists.)

Incident report: formal written report that informs hospital administrators (and the hos-

pital's insurance company) about an incident and that serves as a contemporary factual statement in the event of a lawsuit

Incremental record: record kept according to time and occurrences

Independent practice association (IPA) model HMO: health maintenance organization that contracts with an association of doctors to provide doctor services to its members while the doctors maintain their independent practices

Informed consent: permission obtained from a patient to perform a specific test or procedure after the patient has been fully informed about the test or procedure

Interventions: nursing actions taken to meet a patient's health care needs; should reflect nurse's agreement with the patient on how to meet defined goals or expected outcomes

Joint Commission on Accreditation of Healthcare Organizations (JCAHO): private, nongovernmental agency that establishes guidelines for the operation of hospitals and other health care facilities, conducts accreditation programs and surveys, and encourages the attainment of high standards of institutional medical care, with members that include representatives from the American Medical Association, American College of Physicians, and American College of Surgeons

Katz index: assessment tool used to evaluate a patient's ability to perform the basic functions of bathing, dressing, toileting, transfer, continence, and feeding

Lawton scale: assessment tool used to evaluate a patient's ability to perform relatively complex tasks, such as using a telephone, cooking, managing finances, and taking medications

Learning outcomes: outcomes developed as part of a patient-teaching plan that identify what a patient needs to learn, how you'll teach him, and how you'll evaluate what he's learned

Living will: witnessed document indicating a patient's desire to be allowed to die a natural death, rather than be kept alive by life-sustaining measures; applies to decisions that will be made after a terminally ill patient is incompetent and has no reasonable possibility of recovery

Minimum data set (MDS): standardized assessment tool that must be filled out for every patient admitted to a long-term care facility as mandated by the federal government

North American Nursing Diagnosis Association (NANDA): organization responsible for developing and categorizing nursing diagnoses and examining applications of nursing diagnoses in clinical practice, education, and research

Nursing diagnosis: clinical judgment made by a nurse about a patient's responses to actual or potential health problems or life processes; describes a patient problem that the nurse can legally solve; may apply to families and communities as well as individual patients

Nursing process: systematic approach to identifying a patient's problems and then taking nursing actions to address them; steps include assessing the patient's problems, forming a diagnostic statement, identifying expected outcomes, creating a plan to achieve expected outcomes and solve the patient's problems, implementing the plan or assigning others to implement it, and evaluating the plan's effectiveness

Occurrence reporting: Reporting by doctors, nurses, or other hospital staff of incidents, either when they're observed or shortly after; also called incident reporting

Occurrence screening: identification of adverse events through a review of medical records

Outcome criteria: standards by which measurable goals (outcomes) are objectively evaluated

Outcome documentation: charting that focuses on patient behaviors and responses to nursing care; documents the patient's condition in relation to predetermined outcomes included in the plan of care

Peer review organization (PRO): basic component of a quality improvement program in which the results of health care given to a specific patient population are evaluated according to outcome criteria established by peers of the professionals delivering the care; promoted by professional organizations as a means of maintaining standards of care

Practice guidelines: sequential instructions for treating patients with specific health problems

Preadmission screening annual resident review (PASARR): form used to assess the mental status of a patient before admission to a long-term care facility; required for Medicare or Medicaid reimbursement

Problem-intervention-evaluation (PIE) charting: charting system that organizes patient information according patient's problems; integrates the patient's plan of care into the progress notes in order to simplify the documentation process

Problem-oriented medical record (POMR): method of organizing the medical record; consists of baseline data, a problem list, and a plan of care for each problem

Quality improvement: commitment on the part of a health care facility or several health disciplines to work together to achieve an optimal degree of excellence in the services rendered to every patient (State regulatory and accrediting agencies may require health care facilities to regularly monitor, evaluate, and seek ways to improve the quality of care.)

Resident assessment protocol (RAP): form required by federal mandate for use in long-term care facilities that identifies the patient's primary problems and care needs and documents the existence of a plan of care

Risk management: identification, analysis, evaluation, and elimination or reduction of risks to patients, visitors, or employees; involves loss prevention and control and the handling of all incidents, claims, and other insurance- and litigation-related tasks.

SOAP charting: structured method of recording progress notes in which data is organized into the following categories: Subjective, Objective, Assessment, and Planning

SOAPIE charting: structured method of recording progress notes in which data is organized into the following categories: Subjective, Objective, Assessment, Planning, Implementation, and Evaluation

SOAPIER charting: structured method of recording progress notes in which data is organized into the following categories: Subjective, Objective, Assessment, Planning, Implementation, Evaluation, and Revision

Source-oriented narrative record: method of organizing the medical record in which each discipline records information in a separate section of the medical record

Utilization review: program, initiated by reimbursing agents to maintain control over health care providers, that may focus on length of stay, treatment regimen, validation of tests and procedures, and verification of the use of medical supplies and equipment

Index

i refers to an illustration; t refers to a table

i refers to an illustration; t refers to a table

i refers to an illustration; t refers to a table

i refers to an illustration; t refers to a table

i refers to an illustration; t refers to a table

i refers to an illustration; t refers to a table

i refers to an illustration; t refers to a table